Performance Research is an independent, peer reviewed journal published by Routledge for ARC, a division of the Centre for Performance Research Ltd, an educational charity limited by guarantee, which works with the support of the Arts Council of Wales. Performance Research acknowledges support from the University of Wales, Aberystwyth, De Montfort University and Dartington College of Arts.

Performance Research welcomes responses to the ideas and issues it raises and is keen to consider proposals for articles and submissions. Please address all correspondence to:

Clancy Pegg
Journal Administrator
Performance Research
Market Road
Canton
Cardiff CF5 1QE
Wales, UK

Tel. and Fax: +44 (0) 1 222 388848
Email: post@perfres.demon.co.uk

Performance Research is published three times a year by Routledge, 11 New Fetter Lane, London EC4P 4EE UK A full listing of Routledge journals is available by accessing http://journals.routledge.com

Enquiries concerning subscriptions should be addressed to Routledge Subscriptions Department, North Way, Andover, Hants SP10 5BE, UK
Tel.: +44 (0) 1264 343062   Fax: +44 (0) 1264 343005
For sample copies contact the Subscriptions Department or email: sample.journals@routledge.com

ISSN 1352–8165
© Routledge 1998

Annual subscription rates:
£ (Sterling):   Institution £88   Personal £30
US$:   Institution $140   Personal $45

Members of the Centre for Performance Research (CPR) will receive Performance Research as part of their membership. For further information please contact:

Adam Hayward
Centre for Performance Research
8 Science Park, Aberystwyth
Ceredigion SY23 3AH
Wales, UK

Tel.: + 44(0)1970 622133
Fax: + 44(0) 1970 622132
Email: cprwww@aber.ac.uk

Design: Secondary Modern
Typeset by Type Study, Scarborough, UK
Printed in the UK by Bell & Bain, Glasgow

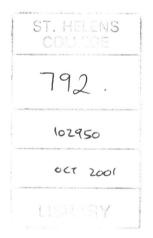

EDITORIAL STATEMENT

Performance Research is a peer reviewed performing arts journal published three times a year. It is international in scope with an emphasis on contemporary European performance. The journal aims to promote a cross-disciplinary exchange of ideas and stimulate discourses surrounding established, experimental, speculative and prospective performance work. Each issue combines thematic and general content from the current field of performance research and practice.

SUBMISSIONS

The editors are interested in encouraging submissions and proposals for forthcoming issues. We welcome proposals using visual, graphic and photographic forms, including photo essays and original artwork for the page, as well as substantial articles and in-depth performance, archive and book reviews. There is no payment for articles except in the case of commissions for which funding might be sought. It is the responsibility of authors to seek permission for all visual and other copyright material.

Proposals may be submitted on one sheet of A4 containing an abstract, proposed word count and description. Unsolicited articles may be submitted for consideration by email attachment, on disk or double spaced in hard copy. Detailed guidelines for preparing text will be sent either on request or on acceptance for publication. Proposals are considered at least nine months before publication.
Proposals and articles, including reviews, should be sent to:

Clancy Pegg, Administrator, Performance Research, Market Road, Cardiff, CF5 1QE, Wales, UK.
Email: post@perfres.demon.co.uk

PLEASE NOTE that proposed submissions do not necessarily have to relate to issue themes. We actively welcome submissions on any area of performance research, practice and scholarship.

FORTHCOMING ISSUES

The next three issues of Performance Research will be entitled *On Ritual* (Autumn 1998), *On Cooking* (Spring 1999) and *On Line* (Summer 1999).

On Ritual will examine a range of performative practices from both the historical and contemporary repertoire. It will explore systematic connections between ritual and theatre, present the work of contemporary artists, and reflect on the role and meaning of ritual for theatrical purposes in the late twentieth century. The issue will also look at ritualism in the interstices of painting, music and theatre, the role of rituals for personal and social identity, and the antithesis of healing rituals and rituals of death.

On Cooking. This issue will explore themes reflected in the overlap between Performance, Food and Cookery. It will look at food in performance and food as performance art; the performative in cookery and its staging in the kitchen and at the table. Articles and artists' pages will develop piquant analogies and correlations between the processes in cooking and performance making. They will give testament to the theatricality of food and speculate on food as a model for theatre: multi-sensory, processual and communal.

On Line. Emerging digital media, information and communications technologies are changing the ways in which we understand and experience time and space, place and body. These developments challenge us to redefine existing strategies and forms of performance, and to create fresh approaches and alternative environments for performance making and composition. *On Line* will explore these changing conditions as they relate to performance practice and discourse. The editors invite materials from individuals and groups involved in exploring territories where emerging technologies and performance overlap and intersect, as well as excavations of the histories of performance and technology.

Volume 3 No. 2. Summer 1998

On Place

* An acetate overlay is provided with this issue for use with pp. 15–18

Performance Research
A Journal of Performing Arts

GENERAL EDITOR
Richard Gough
Artistic Director, Centre for Performance Research and
Senior Research Fellow, University of Wales, Aberystwyth

JOINT EDITORS
Claire MacDonald
Senior Lecturer and Research Fellow, De Montfort
University, Leicester, UK
Ric Allsopp
Founder of Writing Research Associates and Research
Fellow, Dartington College of Arts, Totnes, UK

CONSULTANT EDITOR
Talia Rodgers
Routledge, London, UK

ASSOCIATE EDITORS
Noel Witts
De Montfort University, Leicester, UK
Alan Read
Roehampton Institute, London, UK

GUEST EDITORS: ON PLACE
Mark Minchinton
Victoria University, Melbourne, Australia
David Williams
Victoria Univeristy, Melbourne, Australia

CONTRIBUTING EDITORS
Philip Auslander Georgia Institute of Technology, USA
Günter Berghaus University of Bristol, UK
Rustom Bharucha Writer, Critic and Theoretician, Calcutta, India
Johannes Birringer Northwestern University, Chicago, USA
Dwight Conquergood Northwestern University, Chicago, USA
Scott deLahunta Writing Research Associates, Amsterdam,
Netherlands
Josette Féral University of Quebec, Montreal, Canada
Coco Fusco Tyler School of Art, Philadelphia, USA
Peter Holland The Shakespeare Institute, University of Birmingham,
Stratford-upon-Avon, UK
Nick Kaye University of Warwick, Coventry, UK
Andrea Phillips Freelance Writer and Editor, London, UK
Heike Roms Theatre Researcher, Hamburg, Germany and Cardiff, UK
David Williams Victoria University, Melbourne, Australia
Nicholas Zurbrugg De Montfort University, Leicester, UK

EUROPEAN CORRESPONDENT EDITORS
Knut Ove Arntzen University of Bergen, Norway
Toni Cots Theatre Researcher, Copenhagen, Barcelona and Caracas
Christine Gaigg Freelance Writer and Performer, Vienna, Austria
Emil Hrvatin Director and Dramaturg, Ljubljana, Slovenia
Antonio Fernandez Lera Writer and Journalist, Madrid, Spain
Hans Thies Lehmann Johann Wolfgang Goethe-Universität,
Frankfurt am Main, Germany

ADVISORY BOARD
Eugenio Barba Director, Nordisk Teaterlaboratorium, Holstebro,
Denmark
Brian Catling Ruskin School of Drawing, Oxford University, UK
Enzo Cozzi Royal Holloway, University of London, UK
Norman Frisch Dramaturg and Producer, New York, USA
Peter Hulton Director, Arts Documentation Unit, Exeter, UK
Stephanie Jordan Roehampton Institute, London, UK
Alastair MacLennan University of Ulster, UK
Drew Milne Trinity Hall, Cambridge, UK
Patrice Pavis University of Paris 8, France

ADMINISTRATOR
Clancy Pegg Cardiff, UK

Preface

Both place and placelessness have been very much my experience over the last few months working as 'shadow' editor for this issue 'On Place'. The seeming erasure of distance brought about by digital telecommunications has provided me with a constant sense of vertigo as we put together the contributions for an issue that involved the simultaneous efforts of people in South Africa, London, Arizona, Melbourne, California, Wales and Devon. The apparent absence of some of the traditional attributes of place (separation, distance) brings into focus the importance of the differences of voices, agendas and discourses partly created by the realities of geographical and cultural distance. These differences, brought together in performance and on the page, cut through the insularities of cultural attitudes. Whilst maintaining particularity – a sense of a place within an ongoing debate – they can provide a means to rethink where we (as readers, as participants) are ourselves taking place. I would like to thank the individual contributors for their insights into performance, place and praxis, and not least both guest editors for their time and energy in editing this issue. Mark Minchinton is now busy persuing research on driving as performance, and David Williams has just returned to England after ten years in Australia to take up a post as Professor of Theatre at Dartington College of Arts. *Performance Research* wishes them both well.

Ric Allsopp, editor (East Allington, July 1998)

Frontwords

There is always a place, a tree or grove, in the territory where all the forces come together in a hand-to-hand combat of energies. The earth is this close embrace. This intense centre is simultaneously inside the territory, and outside several territories that converge on it. . . . Inside or out, the territory is linked to this intense centre, which is like the unknown homeland, terrestrial source of all forces friendly and hostile, where everything is decided.

(Deleuze and Guattari 1987: 321)

'Place', with its extended range of generic and metaphorical applications, is an enormously multi-layered and ambiguous term in the English language. And places themselves are constructed and distinguished in many ways. As repositories of public and private memories, for example, 'talismans' of dis/continuity (Etlin 1997: 310 and van den Berg, Walker, Danko, Stafford and

Kemp/Minchinton in this issue). Or in terms of scale, extending in sliding measures from individual bodies – the primary 'place' – to home and community, city, region, nation and globe (see Smith 1993 and Soboslay, Laing, Hill/Paris and Pearlman in this issue). Indeed, places are produced at any and every level of perceived identity and difference: economic, racial, gendered, sexual, religious, climatic, topographic, etc. If space is often conceived as Time's other, then place is enmeshed in contextual histories, (re)produced through praxes.

But what is the place of teletopic actions-at-a-distance, in which our territorial and animal bodies are displaced by the horizonless, gravity-free circuits, flows and sedentary terminals of real-time information technologies? Paul Virilio offers a rather shrill and absolutist vision of a crippling 'grey ecology' of 'dromospheric pollution' that

> attacks the liveliness of the *subject* and the mobility of the *object* by atrophying the *journey* to the point where it becomes needless. A major handicap, resulting both from *the loss of the locomotive body* of the passenger, the tele-viewer, and from the loss of that solid ground, of that vast floor, identity's adventure playground of being in the world.
>
> (Virilio 1997: 33–4; emphases in original)

And what of the universalizing white cube of galleries, the black box of theatres, places deliberately voided of location? Or the con-fusions characteristic of those 'non-places' elaborated in the citationality of contemporary capitalism – shopping malls, airports, hotels, and so on?

> Here in Southern California . . . I can go into the sterile and bizarre setting of a shopping mall to purchase a genuine leather bag, while a group of Mexicans with motors strapped to their backs are blowing away fallen leaves from indoor Australian native trees, while Mozart plays from concealed loudspeakers at a nearby Sushi bar.
>
> (Zutter 1993: 39)

It seems 'there is no there there', to borrow a phrase from Gertrude Stein. And yet all such *utopian* sites, where referentially drained signs of place are dis-located and commodified as pastiche

style for consumption, will inevitably be construed, practised, resisted and inhabited in multiple and contrapuntal ways. As Michel de Certeau has argued, consumption may be productive, in a *poiesis* of 'surreptitious creativities' (de Certeau 1988: xi–xiii). I think of the graffito on a sign at the entrance to Highpoint, one of Melbourne's sprawling malls, the 'High' erased and replaced with a 'No'. Or of the Canberra child who was publicly 'shamed' recently by being paraded through the shopping mall 'scene-of-the-crime' wearing a T-shirt emblazoned with the words 'I am a thief'; within a week, I am told, this sign of stigmatization had been co-opted and undermined as identical T-shirts were printed and worn around Canberra's malls by many others. All places are heterotopias 'really', as many of the contributors to this issue of *Performance Research* attest.

Place is closely interwoven with a network of terms that relate to ownership and its attendant behavioural socius: proper, property, propriety, appropriate. Hélène Cixous's analysis of the imperialist economies of morbidity, which she names *l'Empire du propre* (the Empire of the selfsame), traces this network and its strategies, as does de Certeau:

> A strategy assumes a place that can be circumscribed as proper (*propre*). . . . Political, economic and scientific rationality has been constructed on this strategic model. . . . The 'proper' is a victory of space over time.
>
> (de Certeau 1988: xix)

The unadorned literality of such strategies' repeated enactment in relatively recent history, as erasure-of-difference through reproduction-of-Same, is astounding. Here are two examples that recite an all-too-familiar figure of identity in re-siting the identical figure: in June 1938, the Nazis desecrated and demolished Munich's main synagogue, turning place into the policed and parcelled uniformity of a carpark; and during the Vietnam War, General William Westmoreland declared with some relish that he was going to turn Vietnam itself into a 'parking lot'. Terms related to proper/ty have a particular topicality and discursive gravity in contemporary Australia (my adopted 'home' as an insider-outsider migrant) where the meanings of place and legitimized ownership of these meanings are now more fiercely contested than ever. In what follows, I take 'Australia' – like 'America' or 'Europe' – to be both a geophysical site and a set of ideas or constitutive myths jostling for position.

In traditional Aboriginal cultures in Australia, in which identities are inseparably imbricated in places, one's 'country' constitutes a series of texts, *mappae mundi* of lore/law. Creation myths, sacred teachings, cultural histories and geographies are inscribed on the 'maternal' body of the land itself. Physiographic features record the exploits of totemic ancestors, which may be read, like Braille, and re-animated in the present. 'Here and there they discarded pieces of their body – organs, limbs, hair, lice, skin, nails and teeth which metamorphose into physical features of the landscape' (Mundine 1996: 46): rock formations, trees, river courses, waterholes, and so on. In Pierre Nora's formulation, such interconnected features comprise '*milieux de mémoire*, real environments of memory', rather than '*lieux de mémoire*', isolated monuments (Nora 1989: 7). For journeys through these places, with the narrative song cycles that articulate their numinosity for the initiated, constitute performative re-makings, re-earthings, re-memberings of originary happenings here now, fusing place, body and spirit at the intersection of secular and sacred time. To walk the story is to revisit and rehearse corporeally the itineraries of a tradition that maps the complex interrelatedness of cultural spaces and identities, pasts and possible futures. To walk the story is to privilege the route, to inhabit the space between here and there, between dwelling and travelling, and to respect its 'logic of intensities': an 'eco-logic', the evolutive process of which 'seeks to grasp existence in the very act of its constitution; it is a process of "setting into being"' (Guattari 1989: 136). To walk the story is to attend to landscape as inscape, and to take (a) place in the world.

In an essay entitled 'Teatrum nondum cognitorum' ('Theatre of the not yet known') about the

limits of cartography as representation, Paul Foss proposes a psychogeography of Australia in terms of its early explorers' and colonizers' dis-placed relationships to their spatial environments, and the subsequent cultural impact of their narratives on modern Australians (Foss 1981). Foss describes a constructed 'antipodal space' – the other hemisphere, the place of the other – as being historically defined in terms of void, lack, or absence: a non-place, a *tabula rasa* on which to project anxieties and fantasies. From the moment of so-called discovery, European explorers chose to perceive this 'Great Southern Land' as a place of no visible contents, no inhabitants, no water, no inland seas, no songbirds: a stretch of nothing, a scorched and smouldering vacuum, a place of disappearance, a vanishing-point. *Terra nullius*, they called it, ascribing its features with names that memorialize their own senses of being 'out of place': Mount Misery, Cape Catastrophe, Lake Disappointment and Useless Loop. In such a limbo, there could be 'nothing out there'. Ideal for castaways – or for penal colonies to rid the so-called civilized world of its 'waste'. Imperial History taught Australians to view their island as a 'waste-land', an excess of space, way beyond the comprehension and possessive hunger of the representatives of an expanding empire. You can't possess it, went the story, but it may just possess and consume you – like so many of its early explorers, who entered this lacuna in the assumed order of Harmonious Creation and 'died of landscape' (Stow 1969).

Contemporary Australia is an island continent – a term which in itself, of course, infers both isolation and size – within which urban places still cling to the coastal strips: 'to the outer rim as if ready to depart' (Ireland 1980: 310). For Australia is built around an interior that, through European lenses, remains unplaceable (atopian), unknowable, terrifying, to be kept outside: the 'out-back', the 'dead centre'. Culturally, it seems, many Australians feel obliged to look 'out' rather than 'in', thereby privileging insularity to the detriment of interiority and futurity. As novelist David Ireland wrote in *A Woman of the Future*: 'Australia . . . sits on the comfortable coast of life, where its settled nature is steeped in the past. The future is the greatest problem. The future is at the centre of Australia's problems' (Ireland 1980: 187). In recent years, this central 'void' has been increasingly colonized – by British nuclear test sites, American tracking installations, multinational mining concerns, vast properties – then abandoned to create new wastelands, toxic no-go zones like Maralinga or Wittenoom. Meanwhile the notion of an empty centre of deserts, desertion and desolation stubbornly persists, despite the fact that this is only a *simulacrum* of the void, a construction. Of course countless peoples, cultures, places *do* exist there; it is not empty at all.

> [T]he very habit and faculty that makes apprehensible to us what is known and expected dulls our sensitivity to other forms, even with the most obvious. We must rub our eyes and look again, clear our minds of what we are looking for to see what is there.
>
> (Malouf 1994: 130)

If they remain largely 'unseen', as do Aboriginal peoples and their claims to the places and lives stolen from them for so many on the 'comfortable coast of life', this lack of re-cognition stems from more than blinkered or flawed perception. It relates to a refusal to look in, or behind, to the enduring shadows. To listen to the 'empty space' at the heart, and to apprehend it as a dynamic place for re-reading and rewriting histories and geographies: a theatre of the not yet known, where everything is (to be) decided.

David Williams, guest editor
Melbourne, 24 March 1998

ACKNOWLEDGEMENT

The guest editors would like to thank the following for their help in the preparation of 'On Place': Richard Murphet, Jude Walton, and in particular Ric Allsopp and Clancy Pegg; and all those who sent contributions for which we could find no place here.

REFERENCES

de Certeau, Michel (1988) *The Practice of Everyday Life*, Berkeley: University of California Press.

Deleuze, Gilles and Guattari, Félix (1987) *A Thousand Plateaus: Capitalism and Schizophrenia*, trans. Brian Massumi, Minneapolis and London: University of Minnesota Press.

Etlin, Richard A. (1997) 'Space, stone and spirit: the meaning of place', in S. Golding (ed.) *The Eight Technologies of Otherness*, London and New York: Routledge.

Foss, Paul (1981) 'Teatrum nondum cognitorum', *The Foreign Bodies Papers*, Sydney: Local Consumption Papers, Sydney University.

Guattari, Félix (1989) 'The Three Ecologies', trans. Chris Turner, *New Formations* 8 (Summer).

Ireland, David (1980) *A Woman of the Future*, Harmondsworth, Mx: Penguin.

Malouf, David (1994) *Remembering Babylon*, London: Vintage.

Mundine, Djon (1996) '. . . Without land we are nothing. Without land we are a lost people . . .', in V. Somerset (ed.) *Spirit + Place: Art in Australia 1861–1996*, Sydney: Museum of Contemporary Art.

Nora, Pierre (1989) 'Between memory and history: les lieux de mémoire', *Representations* 26.

Smith, Neil (1993) 'Homeless/global: scaling places', in J. Bird, B. Curtis, T. Putnam, G. Robertson and L. Tickner (eds) *Mapping the Futures: Local Cultures, Global Change*, London and New York: Routledge.

Stow, Randolph (1969) 'The singing bones', in *A Counterfeit Silence*, Sydney: Angus & Robertson.

Virilio, Paul (1997) *Open Sky*, trans. Julie Rose, London: Verso.

Zutter, Jorg (1993) 'Interview with Bill Viola', *Art and Design* 31 (London): 'World Wide Video'.

SMALLNESS AND INFINITY
Living, writing, travelling,
making [in] the world

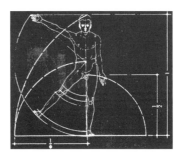

*Zsuzsanna Soboslay Moore is a performance-maker who has taught her own bodytuning method across the eastern states of Australia, and trained in various theatrical traditions including shamanic dance. In this article she discusses two of her performance works: **the awakenings project**, a movement opera with new text which took the German play* Spring Awakening *as its springboard, and **Landscape Jazz,** an ecological cross-form improvisation process she has developed over several years.* **awakenings** *premiered in Sydney in August 1997;* **Burn,** *the second of the three interactions in* **Landscape Jazz,** *was improvised in the Sutherland National Park, Sydney, in May 1996.*

It's suddenly realizing that the world is big, the universe is infinite and we have so little say in it. The Germans would call [the feeling] *Weltschmerz,* **world-pain. One feels the vanity of it all. The universal meaning of one's life can only be experienced as emptiness. And the peculiar thing is that we have no choice but to accept it; and yet we cannot**.

Interview: Jan Sedivka, violinist and '60s immigrant, Master Resident at University of Tasmania, with Louise Oxley, *Siglo* 6 (Tasmania, 1996): 48–9.

... it dawned on me that this is not a new country, it's the oldest country. It seems to be unchangeable because it's been so long there.... It gives us somehow our identity through its enormity. It's not that we give it the identity. The idea that we came to conquer Australia is somehow silly. This realization made me open my eyes a little bit, and now I not only feel at home, but rather humble, I must say.

Jan Sedivka, ibid.: 52.

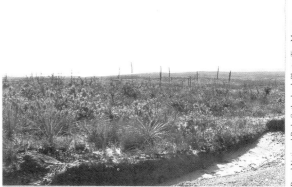

Royal National Park Sutherland Photo: Tim Moore

Tracking: listening to history, memory and time.
Cell memory: documenting coinhabitants.
Excavation: resurrection, reinhabitation.
Territory/ownership: what training aspires to. Who owns it.

1950—AWASH

They travelled the sea in a migration awash with vomit and crying children. Some of the refugees had not seen a toilet bowl before, and used them as vanity-units. The hull festered with people who for three months had no place to wash themselves. They were Magyars, Serbs, Russians, Poles; no one spoke each other's language. My mother escaped to surface duties, saved from this dungeon by her knowledge of English. The sea captain employed her to type his official naval letters home.

They arrived, most of them, to camps and canning factories. Hot summer bush and unheated icy winters on long dry treeless plains. They slept under tin roofs, and ate God knows what—mostly remnants from the canneries. The country hardly welcomed them: they were ordered to speak English in the streets, on trams, the gift horse's teeth knocked out of its head countless times. My mother never spoke much of her experiences, only expressed gratitude for a country which took her away from the spiritual and physical deprivations and political chaos of back home. Although, it's hard to know exactly what she lost: to this day, she speaks as if the worst wound on her country was the blowing up of bridges across the Danube in the Nazi retreat of '45, and the raising of hammer and sickle on top of the Houses of Parliament that still are Budapest's pride. My father's story is another matter: perhaps the experience of the Russian Front was so unspeakable that it marked the death of his former life to which he never again referred. Neither ever particularly wanted gifts of books written in their native tongue. As a child, I used to wonder why.

Slowly they regained some of their familiars, though mostly they did not. A landscape full of new tastes and smells, the occasional excitement of finding poppy-seeds or well-smoked ham. Lusts and tastes of association breed in the blood: to this day, certain smoky-pink and wood-panelled restaurants still trigger in me a desire for cake, coffee and Europe I don't otherwise have. The jumping of landscape across generations is phenomenal; perhaps there's a tastebud DNA. This smell, that timbre, that rise of the mountain; fragments shored, perhaps, against the ruins of the heart. Or perhaps the heart is a prism of fragile glass, catching old illusions. Whatever, the sensations are real, and remain.

When we talk about landscape, it's not abstract: a copse of trees, the roar of wind, moistness like a halo round the skin, affecting and effecting us. When you turn the corner, your breathing changes.The new vista sets up a different correspondence. The body and landscape write letters to each other.

In May I was in Turkey—quite close enough to the 'home country' I somehow fear setting my foot into. Traditionally, the Turks are the bloody so-and-so's the Hungarians kept in their pockets like a steam-ironed clipping from a wound. In Turkey, however, I felt reciprocal animosities. They have their own, perhaps more crumpled, summaries.

Yet the similarities! Their nationhood, their person-hoods written in the pavements, rivers and walls. Where the museums become too cramped, history is tossed into the streets—feet, arms, half-faces chiselled in stone—and imbued in these antiquities is a similar pride in their longevity, the pride of a race which has fought, conquered, been conquered—and holds its grudges: *This limb comes from the ruins of Ephesus; the British have all the rest.* I knew I was in Europe when I tasted that spiced coffee-scented

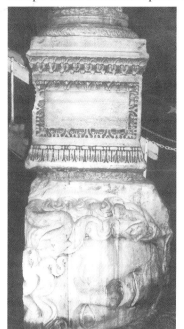

grudge. We copped it, being tourists: fair game on the circuit of give and take and steal and give again. This land shored with its ancient battle-lines.

Column Medusa, Istanbul.
Photo: Tim Moore

And my own shoreline? Compressed in my ribs: unspecified histories, bottled memories, the battles of families and empires, brewed in a new country bordered only by the sea, within the complacency of treelined suburbs and starched pinafores . . .

A decade ago, I wrote a piece about a Russian composer of this century, mainly sourced from his music and a biography. I am astonished how much I knew about his historical experience: the spilt blood on the streets, the sound of marching boots, the puffery of armies. How do I know this? How has my skin absorbed a landscape in which I've never been, unless landscape is carried through words, sounds, paintings, gestures, and all the unspokens you share with people as you climb (or fail) the same mountains together. Unless history, memory themselves are landscapes that draw the world like a pencil, adding their own colours (perhaps more real than the photograph) and remap, *prodding, provoking and preventing* the remaking of the world?

PROD
The Shaman[1] dances.
Melbourne, 1993 Tokyo, 1995

She becomes peacock
baby letcher tree
newspaper-in-wind
cicada shell.
She teaches,
feeding the body
with images:
Light falling on a leaf. Photosynthesis.

The mountain
rises beside her, there is dust
in her tail;
the memory of animal
within her changing the
bite and heat of air.

This is
belonging, and
loss. She is
everything, and alone. It is
elationary,
evolutionary . . . and
frightening.

to work as if you are a network of nerves
to work with uncertainty
to change internal speed, to walk through walls
to consider the condition of space around you as
substance,
affected by your transformation.

Become vibration

PROVOKE

Honshu, 1995. Another tremor.
They live on a fault line. The earth
shakes regularly, and on some days
with particular violence. *What*
tremor? I feel no tremor.
But the earth lifted and shook
the building like a child would
an errant bear.

Some questions
are too much. Even the
borderliners,   the artists
                                                          and hobos,
                                          blink as if they have
                              not heard—
                        [because on
                  some level,   we
            have to keep our footing]

VATERLAND

The Wall trips itself up on the pavement; gets a bit too drunk to stand . . . .

Timothy Garton Ash (1990) writes of being present in '89 at the fall of the Berlin Wall. Funny word, *fall*, to describe something pulled down by the collected and condensed will of so many people. Their shoulders are the ramparts, their bursting throats the arrows. What he remembers of the crowd moving from East to West was the simplicity of their actions: a walk, a look, a shop, perhaps for fruit, and their return. But what they called out for in the streets, what they wanted, was not just the untrammelled view, a glimpse of a wealthier world, but *reunification*: DEUTSCHLAND, EINIG VATERLAND. One Germany, one Fatherland.[2]

That's what we lose, in war: our men, our father-place, our god. Our sense of a largeness that contains us. This feeling, *Weltschmerz,* is the subject of huge pain.

I keep having dreams of a child who is vomiting. *She has been looking for her father.* In life, I spent many years being this child. I lost my father when I was twelve. About this, I still do not know my fury. But I too have lost my country: *she vomits. She has been looking for her father.* [It has taken many years to put down my heels.] Nothing in our history-books—the tales of battlegrounds drawn, possessed, and redrawn—teaches that *to be in place is to be humble.*

I can own a coffee-pot, silver, paintings, jewels; somewhere in Hungary we have a castle, rambling and rumbling, no doubt, down a sovereign hill. Useless. *In performance I own nothing.* My grandmother, a later immigrant, stuffed her horsehair chair with memories, hoarding her silvers and Chippendales in stories that she sat in, sat on, cloaked around herself like the Emperor's Clothes. She believed in her tailors, and the cobblers whose narrow shoes deformed her feet for ever; indeed her whole life, up until the war, had been the making concrete of those tailorings. The war was the child that laughed at her, decimating the fantastic silks in which she lived. In her migration, only the stories survived, packed in walnut shells. We had no concrete inheritance, only the remnant pride. She never went exploring from the perch of her horsehair, and hated her adoptive land until the day she died.

My parents refused her nostalgia, quietly numbing their bones, deterring their own shadows. That effort was immense; yet they seemed to prefer it to remounting their own stories. We lived in a tug-of-war between negation and desire in a new land we hardly had the space to hear.

PREVENT

1985: I take my mother into the heart of ancient Western Sydney mangroves. We wanted to see the new park, commemorated for the Bicentennial [so young a celebration]. The mangroves' muscled arms dipped and drank the slimy waters of the billabong as if their thirst were insatiable. Hard, strong, dry-boned, this landscape made her cringe as she walked. *Call this beautiful?* she spat, clambering along the walkway as if those broad arms, at any step, might take her.

Compared to her Europe, this territory lacked the greenery, shrubbery, the ordered and elegant undulating folds of harvest patchworks stitched with chestnuts and elms. I think the root systems were too much – a threat, like the bare legs of a warrior advancing. But one which couldn't care less if we were there or not. The War, by contrast, must have been intimate: bombs shattering the sandstones they loved, and chandeliers, bodies bundled during air-raids against dank wine-cellar walls, contending with hunger and old men's snores. Could such a war make sense in a different landscape? Can you fight the same way for mangroves?—The fight is something different here: survival, defence, what is of value, are not on the same terms . . .

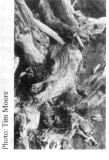

Photo: Tim Moore

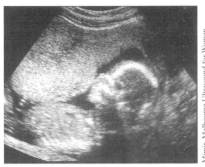

In performance, there cannot be an off-limits zone

Mimir, Melbourne Ultrasound for Women

ZERO

1997: I see the Hamburg Schauspielhaus production of *Stunde Null*.[3] A mayhem of guilt-ridden denials, recounting the point in German post-war history from which their historical world was supposedly new-born. There are eight suited men who sleep on camp-beds, recite the future, suckle at the teats of Matron Zero Hour as if this were the myth-making of a new Rome. Imagine: all these corpulent bodies saying this is their Day One. As if nothing has fed them to this corpulence.[You can feel the hiccough, the teetering, the imbalance, as the shadowed half of the world, sawn off, begins to fall.] So history, night, childhoood, no longer come round to invade the day. Hard to feel a future then, if the world no longer turns....

THE BLACKBOARD SPEAKS:

And I will tell you a story about three men
whose heads lie in their graves
visited only by their wives . . . .
peeled off from memory
like the quarter of an orange
a segment remembered, perhaps, where he liked
potatoes or was kind to the cat

And these quarter men with their ties
dividing the carapace between
left and right, bound and tied,
mouthing words without sound
[There is a half of your life left to live
Where is the the rest of it]
like the child playing hopscotch on the square
          1, 2, buckle my shoe
          3, 4, – forget the rest;
---all it can know
is its father's skull,
carried in its pocket,
its mother's heart written in the
stone it
throws on to the square . . . . .
          . . . Stop counting
          [*Awakenings*, I (i)]

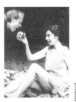

Awakenings. Photos: Paula Sammut

QUICKENING

[1] *Spring Awakening* is a play about children confused between their coming to awareness [blossoming, burgeoning, exploring, daring to show their hearts in the world] and the order of axemen who try to bring the saplings into line. This is Germany in 1892; a small town, the play an *agon* between repression and sensuality, civil and barbarian blood. In *Awakenings*, I reworked the spirit of the text from the perch of the daughter of immigrants who shared a similar *mythos* and cultural background. Someone who heard the music in their heads, felt the sacred buildings behind the unspoken wave of hands, the prejudices, the inheritances, a European sense of borderlines.

I called on shapings in the original playtext which matched more silent shapings of my own: landscapes of memory, devastation, silence, laughter, grape harvests, bulls'-blood wine . . . .

SCHOOLTEACHER (whilst BOY recites a lesson)
The brain of a monkey.
The soul of an ass.
The body of an angel.
Again!!
The smell of dust, and a rose, luscious
luscious at night.
Again, you dumkopf!!
--Nein!
Take him down!

I called forth the other dimension: the body's uncharted maps, the other parts crying in our sleep, winking in our dreams, that wake you slowly with their singing, 'after the Martians have been with you, waking and hearing them in your mind':

This is your heart.
I took it from you.
I took it so you would never get
the chance to feel it beating.
Your own blood, beating . . .

I stole it three
times: —the first: when you were a knight,
          in the grand court that failed. Arthur's playpen; the king in
          tatters like a baby who could not grow
       —the second, when you were a squirming girl crying
          in the reeds, looking for your brothers
       —the third
          when you went out buying peanuts for supper, because you thought I was
          hungry. (laughs)
This is your
heart.   Sit up in the
tree, waiting for me to throw it
high enough to touch you . . .

This is the body's tune, its rebellions, its own knowings. They perhaps are inarticulate, because they have never known their shape. But their potential to speak is waiting to be mined.

Silence holds power for the generals at the border-guard who own the frontiers of the world. Or, it holds the new mapping, the patchwork waiting to be rearranged . . . .

I have seen marsupials at a zoo paralysed by the memory of an electric fence from a distance of twenty yards. Their sensors, facing the fence, know not to feel in that direction.

This is perching, no-land. This is not-feeling, the coagulation of a scar. This is a place where under the surface, a thick coffee brews. This is the place trying not to explode. *Perhaps The Wall did 'fall', with the pressure of this in its stones . . . .*

But the place of renewal is not lamentation . . .

THE GINGER TREE [Finale]
(voice of an older woman)

The ginger tree has seen everything.
The ginger tree has seen it all.
The ginger tree has had its roots sat on by children.
Children have grown through the roots
and touched its navel as it climbed, relishing
the juice from the ground.
It let the children know its secrets
at the foot of the tree
the ginger house
no crumbs to lead them into the furnace
just letting them be there
at the ginger tree
with its roots swelling for the juices to come
from the ground up through its navel
and spread
and talk to the sun

a bit of shade
(*she turns*)
for the chocolate child
a bit of sharp edge
(*she turns*)
for the lemon child

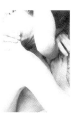
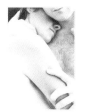
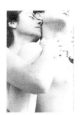
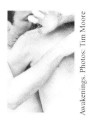

Awakenings. Photos: Tim Moore

and they all come together in ginger root
with its circles
and its skin
and the bite of its taste
knowing sweetness and sour
their tongues knowing
the edge of the bite of its taste
how old it is
how long it has taken to grow
and how easily . . .

*She begins to recede and wither as he
proceeds, inching forward like a baby with its
arms open, hopeful, forehead aglow*

parts die
and come back
feeding the lips of something else
a worm perhaps which would crawl into a skull
and talk to Hamlet, or Ophelia.
Who knows who Ophelia talked to once she
was gone?

Hear the lullaby
the lullaby in the water
telling the ginger its
time was to give way

and the children had to find
another trunk to play with
maybe their own
grow their own roots
because the ginger with its knobbles and
circles and skin
had gone

— became a story
that drew back

and whispered and wavered behind

and left them to go forward, and find
the pond where the reeds danced
because that was their age now:
to dance, letting the petals fall from their skirt
to dance, letting the shawl fall from their breasts
so that they would know each other
the curves of their skin
the pulse of the heart
the pomegranate seed, red rind,
the shape of the lip of pomegranate flesh around
the new thing to be born.

LIGHTS FADE.
THEY CONTINUE.

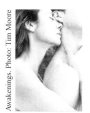

Awakenings. Photo: Tim Moore

[2] LANDSCAPE JAZZ

PROPOSAL: PARATAXES—DISCARDS. [DANCING THE CITY]
A proposition for 3 interactions in 3 sites:

1) Yelp, at the R.S.P.C.A. pound in Yagoona, Sydney
2) Burn, Sutherland National Park (recently burnt by bushfires)
3) Compendium, Studio Space (unrealized)

PARATAXES—SUBJECT:
The phenomenon of the discard, discarding, being lost or being thrown out
(of place; memory; migration, forced exile; penal resettlement; abandonment
[of childhood,puppies, youth, responsibility; coming of age];
—and the discard's residues (gestures towards Homebush Bay and the
chemical-contaminated Olympic site)

Abandonment of old for new (old country for new; old architecture for new;
old lover for new lover; memory vs. future];
Incarnation; re-incarnation and old bones . . . . .
Arson (what is burnt; what is remembered, what returns; what heals itself and grows again);
Architecture: What hovers in memory; what is reconstructed out of incomplete desires.
Voices of the perpetrator and the perpetrated upon.
The urge to (re)build: a subset of a growth force?

STRUCTURES OF COLLABORATION:
                    oppositional (denial of history)
                    empathetic   (individualized collusion)
                    unifying   (construction of future)

Performers: Tess de Quincey, Stuart Lynch, Michael Askill, Zsuzsanna Soboslay.

In May, 1996, de Quincey/Lynch invited
collaborations across Sydney to see if they could
dance it. One hundred in a month: a compression, a
topographing of diverse spaces and activities. I set up
a framework to involve the three of us and Michael
Askill, a percussionist with whom I'd workshopped six
months before.

Sutherland National Park is a bushy footstep to
Sydney's southern sprawl. Its aridity neither embraces
nor comforts; its horizon offers scratchiness and
sunburn. On this morning, gentle-whipping winds
scrub our skins. Fire scorched its tracks five months
before we arrive.

We drive to the firegates in borrowed Holden V8s,
trolley a wheelbarrow full of instruments across the
fire trail, until it sticks in sludge. We carry the drums,
clackers and bells gingerly across an anteater's path.

Our set-up is slow. *How can you time the wind?* A
television crew impatiently nose into armpit-crannies
for close-ups. 'I haven't begun yet', Stuart hisses.
They are admirable, this crew: they simply cannot be
embarrassed. Tess hums on a rock; they traipse and
talk, answer mobile phones.

My fingers tune Michael's body as he works,
reminding sluggish elements of him to respond. Right
ribcage; more warmth in the throat. Although his
fingers drum, I can tell which other parts of him have
become dead zones. Touch immediately opens up a
slightly more...*infected* sound, as if reminding his
body that our feet also dance through him. As if the
inspiration for sound falls into flesh like a rock which
ripples out through water.

Within an hour, the horizon sits in Michael's ribcage.
He is working from the fullest sensing space. When
this happens, something in the scrub itself is released
and begins to walk. Heat from a rock; a bush's secret
dancing. Something in the scrub asks my body to
become part of the shapes changing. I am called to
embrace a bush—or does it cradle me? We rock
together, the rock coming from water sucked at its
roots. Stuart seems to be croaking for a door to open;
Tess is pacing. Our faces mesh with trees.

There is an acute dialectic between this more abstract
state and that of being human. I expand into a
different sense of time, altering vibrations. This is the
place of landforms dividing. There is elation—at the
earth's opening; reconciliation—that the human
knows it, yet is different from it, more solid and more
temporary. I feel my body, my legs, distinct, yet my
belly expands like the earth's core. Something in me
forgives—I can't quite say what. Perhaps the fear of
my own breathing.

At the end of two hours, we all sense completion—
the earth tucking under, rounding off, or in, closing
the magic of its opening. Michael is beaming as his
hand completes the drum; Tess is quiet somewhere to
the side. No one has cued anyone else to stop; Stuart,
who had slowed in before, sits smiling.

THERE IS a map of sensing, knowing, *and an
awareness of the senses' partiality.* There is the third
term: an awareness that, around the corner, is
something beyond your knowing. There is something
in the silence, in the quiet of the unspoken, the still
numb.

Where the battalions have tied you down, *tickle their release . . .*

And in their release is . . . a placelessness; neither *Vaterland,* nor Zero, but a holding, hovering, which equals but does not annihilate our identities. This place is luminous: both magnificent and intimate, a god swinging through, by means of our sensors. *This god has tongues.*

Your speech forms in the cavities of my body. I listen to your substance, your winds, your resistances and your bones.

The work speaks of and from the land, catches the weeping of the mountains, the massacres in the trees. There is memory in the topography of the plains, the knowing a tree has of its neighbour, a document in its rings. Perhaps it shared water in these years, broke a path together with another, shared a loss. Traces of sabotage and love rubbed alongside the landscape's markings like animal spoor. Trees have an endless patience; their sensing exists whether or not we accompany them. *Sentience* is not just the discovery of hard-line scientists gone soft in old age.

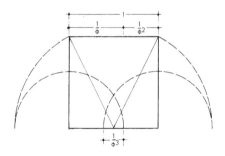

The exterior of a form is produced from its interior: it comes from the centre.
The black produces the white, and vice versa.
A non-absolute edge; a line promising departure
from it
[Kasimir Malevich, in praise of the Square]

The eye resides within the emanation

Is it too much to say *we* do this? That the greatest self-respect we could have is to be equal to this hearing, to know we *co-respond?* Mathematics is emotion and shape has speed and sound. This is our

ordinary madness, a place of knowing and not-knowing. Who's definitely on First Base, What's on Second . . . . . *I Don't Know's on Third.* Not knowing is not chaos, but the place of remaking, hovering until we find the new pattern that coheres.

Thought speaks before it touches breath
The coming-into-being is contiguous with the state from which it comes
The minutest register 'on voice' can move a mountain.
This is how the mountain comes to speak, or dance. We are all vibration.

[TO] DRAW [IN]

At the heart of landscape is geometry—the art of perceiving the underlying nature of proportions and relationship in the world. Interestingly, in ancient Greece, geometry was attributed to the feminine—*an intuitive*

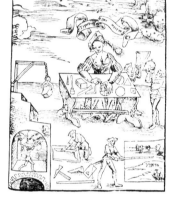

synthesizing, a creative yet exact activity of mind (Lawlor, 1982).

Sometimes, I do everything to avoid hearing what my body is trying to speak, as if it were some monster which disagrees with the order of the world. Whose order? *I am a traveller, a journeyman, a shapeshifter; none of my components fit on supermarket shelves.* Only the barest of landscapes force us to match and learn: that we are equal to the valley, to the hill, to the forces of renewal and decay which move and break and re-form the earth.

I contemplate the aspects in which numerous lives surround a human being . . . . Not only the living but also the dead surround him. I do not know if I dance . . . or deepen my understanding of 'living'. Neither is the case, or both are the case. I dance to cherish life. I practice dance in such a state inbetween.

(Kazuo Ohno, *Butoh Notation,* 1992)

Notes

1 Yoko Ashikawa, one of the original troupe to dance with Tatsumi Hijikata in Japan. At the times mentioned, she was the senior choreographer/teacher with Tomoe Shizune and Hakutobo Theatre Co., Japan.

2 Garton Ash 1990: 71.

3 Deutsches Schauspielhaus, Hamburg. Director: Christophe Marthaler; dramaturg: Stefanie Carp. London LIFT Festival, Queen Elizabeth Hall, Southbank, June 1997

Picture credits:

p.1, Albrecht Dürer, canon figure, in Lawlor 1982: 59.

p.3, 'The Arteries', from Diderot, *L'Encyclopédie ou Dictionnaire raisonné des sciences, des arts et des métiers* (1765) in Feher 1989: 452.

pp.5,6, SHE: Zsuzsanna Soboslay; HE: Benjamin Howes.

p.8, 'The Holy Trinity': 1 = God; 1/pi = the Holy Spirit; 1/pi squared = the Son; in Lawlor 1982: 63.

p.8, G. Reich, 'Margarita Philosophica' (Basle, 1583), in Lawlor 1982: 17.

p.9, Robert Fludd, 'The Pythagorean Triad', *Philosophia sacra et vere Christiana Seu Meteorologia Cosmica,* (Frankfurt: Occicina Bryana, 1626), in Godwin 1979: 31.

References

Bois, Yves-Alain (1987) 'Malevich, the square, degree zero', trans. Frieda Riggs, *On the Beach* 11 (Winter): 17–26.

Feher, Michel (1989), *Zone: Fragments for a History of the Human Body,* Pt III, 'Mapping the Body', by Mark Kidel and Susan Rowe-Leete, New York: Urzone, 448–69.

Garton Ash, Timothy (1990) *We the People–The Revolution of '89,* Cambridge: Granta, pp. 61–77.

Godwin, Jocelyn (1979) *Robert Fludd,* London: Shambala.

Lawlor, Robert (1982) *Sacred Geometry: Philosophy and Practice,* London: Thames & Hudson.

Ohno, Kazuo (1991) 'To cherish life', Interview with Torikoshi Q, *Butoh Bilingual Journal* 1 (Nikutaemo, Spring): 12–13.

Wedekind, Frank (1977) *Spring Awakening* trans. Tom Osborne, London: Calder.

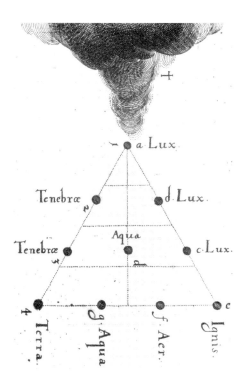

Memorials without Facts

Clive van den Berg

The images used come from an installation called Memorial Without Facts, first made in Johannesburg for an exhibition entitled 'Purity and Danger', curated by Penny Siopis. The installation comprised film, sound, grass, stones, wood and oxides. Many of the images are stills from the film. Most of the footage is original, intercut with historical stills taken from Boer War archives.

Every year, or at least when we could afford it, the family would travel to 'the coast' for a holiday. The coast was in South Africa several thousand miles away. We stayed in a town called Luanshya on the Zambian copper belt. The trip would take several days with stops at various family members along the way. There was Auntie Audrey in Bulawayo. She and her family stayed in Llewellyn Barracks where Uncle Don was a NCO. One of my cousins related how Don had chased Audrey out of the house with a raised spear in his hand. After another night on the road with a stop at Tzaneen we would arrive in Johannesburg to stay with Uncle Allan in a municipal compound next to Soweto. Then it would be on to Auntie Thelma in Dundee where she and Uncle Tommy owned a foundry which made machinery for the coal mines nearby. She always gave us exorbitant amounts of pocket money so we looked forward to that stop most of all. Finally we would reach the coast with both my brother and I anticipating every haze on the horizon as the sea. We would stay for a few weeks and then do the journey in reverse. Those trips taught me something about interior and edge.

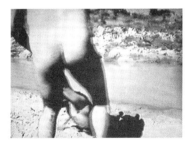

Why were we compelled to holiday only at the edge of the continent?

For these treks we were woken very early. In the dark we would be dressed in khaki shorts and shirts to witness the last-minute packing. Finally it would be time to get into the back seat of the car together with blankets, large packets of 'chips', sweets, and possibly some kind of game, or was that my imagination? I do remember with absolute clarity the feel of chip fragments pinching into the back of my legs. At some point during one of our stops we would sweep the bits out of the car with a thick tartan blanket. This never quite worked and the whole journey would be punctuated with the sharp pain of hardened crisp now embedded in the weave of the rug, pushing into tender skin.

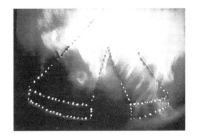

From my position on the back seat of our winged Opel, pink, cream and chrome, I would gaze out of the window at the bush. I could not

Performance Research 3(2), pp.10-14 © Routledge 1998

call it the landscape. I didn't know such a grand word then, although I knew the look of what was proper in the land from books I was given. The bush had none of the comfort and arranged harmony that those picture templates had, none of the sense that history had been covered over with a layer of structured and productive decorum. Rather, it was, for me at least, a jumble of seemingly chaotic yet compelling clues which I tried to decipher, though not yet knowing the questions. For my parents I think it represented something alien. It had as yet no order, certainly no order that could make us holiday there in the interior. It was the bush that we were escaping, something to pass through in between those places that approximated a notion of what was 'civilized'. This bush had not been formed according to the model that the illustrators of those books had used.

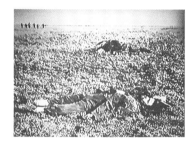

Yet my model was that bush, and I knew it more powerfully than anything that books could give me. I knew it through my skin, the red earth that I made into mud and formed into figures and houses that squelched between my wide-gapped toes in such an orgy of anal pleasure. My parents avoided the 'untamed' bush and sought instead the bowling-green or the club, that essential of even the most modest colonial life. In doing so they avoided the possibility that there was another history in that landscape. These were the things that I sought out. I thrilled to the faintest sight of the past; a piece of a mud wall or a depression in the ground, would excite in me a sense that there was another way of being, that lives perhaps different to mine had been lived out on this land. It was in the medium of space that I first realized that there were other possible conceptions of political and social norms. This was a romantic notion for a child but these motivations and yearnings have persisted in one way or another, linked inextricably with and developing simultaneously to a realization of a sexual identity that was alien to most, or, for all I knew then, to everyone, around me. This fragment of a political realization was the prism through which I recognized the imbrication of space, history and identity.

Yet for me then, and often enough now, I didn't know the 'truth' of the history that I sensed – or rather the history that I had a need for. It was in the landscape that I first realized the comfort of projecting, the importance of the imagination for the creation of an internal political realm in the absence of an external echo of desire. It was precisely because the landscape didn't conform to any model I had received that it became the site of my imaginings and the prompt for desire.

Now I imagine in two directions. Sometimes these imaginings intersect and sometimes they exist more or less parallel to each other.

I am aroused by battle sites, particularly the nineteenth-century battle sites of my home, South Africa. In trying to understand this quiet thrill in my body, the vibrations so akin to sexual excitement, I knew that it was something to do with the emptiness of the space, its simultaneous lack of inscription and over inscription, its burdens of history and abandonment, a kind of forlornness that came with a promise. It is in these places that there seemed to me to be a possibility for another reading of space. It was precisely there, walking amongst the whitewashed, falling-down cairns, along the tops of shallow mounds that demarcated a trench, a mass grave, or both – there, beside, between and on the tokens meant to memorialize the verities of state and family – that I felt the presence of their opposite, the suppressed and tabooed. It was there that I sensed that there was another way, and it was thrilling, this smell of the opposite. In the presence of all these boundaries, the lines of territory, strictures imposed on the body, limits of desire . . . it was there that I felt their inverse.

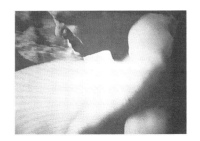

Yet in none of these experiences did I have any facts. Mostly I still don't. I had to trust the divining rod of my sex. I like to think that men loved, fucked, as well as killed each other there. I like to think that there was something in those circumstances that overcame taboos, but it is not really important for me to know; or rather this knowing is not the same as having, or needing, proof. This history was not written, and if it was, it was in terms of a legal documentation of perversion and punishment expressed in the language of the state. What legal documentation confirms is oppression, it rarely gives insight to the more slippery area of suppressed desire. There have been no direct references to same-sex oppression before the Truth and Reconciliation Commission (TRC), a fact which is telling; but there have been narratives of torture that contain repressed references to sex between men – desire as a boil on the skin, expressed as abuse. For example, there is an account of a notorious apartheid torturer who used to force a broomstick up the anus of his victims. Of all the abuses that he freely admits to before the commission, this is the one for which he invokes amnesia. One wonders why? For any of the abuses that were attributable to racism, he sings, but not for those that might have had another impulse. Our archives contain other references to same-sex activity and it is important that we recuperate these documents, but they are only a fragment of the story. These narratives of censure and complaint can't fill in the more speculative realm of desire, the realm of things differently formed. To write only the history of state oppression, the humiliations and tortures suffered by those who loved the same sex, is to ignore another part of this story.

Does that matter, this lack of documented certainties? Not for me . . . or rather, only somewhat. It was enough for me to have found these places that provoke speculation of interior lives.

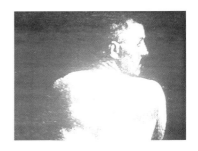

So in order to reform memory according to a different, mostly unwritten schema, I develop visual narratives or conditions of looking that attempt to fill in some of the gaps. To probe those fugitive excesses of history and memory that I first sensed as a child in the back seat of a car driving through the African bush, I make works that I have titled

'Memorials without Facts'. In them I try to insinuate that much more is needed for the recuperation of a nation's memory than the confessions and revelations currently being told to the TRC. I don't in any way wish to undermine or demean those narratives. A very important process is currently being played out in South Africa, but it is always going to be a fragment of the story – not just because only some of the people affected by apartheid will speak, or are able to speak. It is rather that the parameters of what should be legitimated still happen largely within hetero-sexist boundaries.

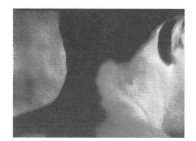

It is important for me that other largely unremarked history is imagined on the land. So many of our narratives of belonging, whether in the form of folk-songs, poetry, or indeed official memorials, use the land as their central motif. Underpinning many of these narratives is a figure of the dutiful man, imaged on the sites of battle, those fissures of terrain that are another way of demarcating the nation. I appropriate sites venerated as proof of what the masculine body should 'properly' be used for, as places to figure a different usage of the body. I make these images as being other than the confirmation of 'productive' action, not the gains of a masculinist energy in the sacrifice for a cause, but rather as subjects that prompt investigation into some alternative life, I suppose a kind of Foucaldian heterotopia. This gives me the licence to memorialize in a different language, and to define purpose in a different way. The memorials that have been erected in our land are meant to provide the evidence that it was all worth it . . . the whole grubby struggle for power and possession that is our history. The need to prove and to justify purpose has dominated our definitions of memory. The contradictions of that history are what presently define what is legitimate for the nation to mourn and memorialize. The love or lust between men and the implications of those states are definitely outside those boundaries. Yet they are interconnected – repression by race and repression by sexual orientation are part and parcel of the same purpose. Neither of these histories has had any official status except in the annals of what was perverse or otherwise unacceptable. The TRC is filling in some of the absences but there is much that is never going to be known. For many in South Africa, not knowing is deeply traumatic and the absence of memorials and relics makes incomplete our transition to the future.

We are currently witnessing confessions from some of the apartheid's most notorious torturers. There are accounts of bodies being blown apart, of bodies being burned to ashes, of bodies being mutilated before death, of bodies being poisoned, of bodies abused and more. In almost all of these accounts the bodies were never recovered. In addition to these lost places of death and abuse there were others where loves, illicit and punishable, were enacted. Sometimes sites can be identified, a piece of land or patch of water that shows no ostensible

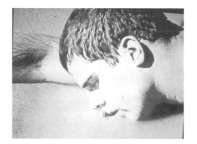

signs of what happened there. A pile of ash, all that remained of a body thrown into a powerful, swiftly moving river, is quickly absorbed. These events for ever intangible are part of our legacy of lives unmemorialized. The need to know where a loved one has been killed and buried, or the fate of the body, is one of the constant refrains heard from the families of victims addressing the TRC. The recentness of these events lends urgency to these needs. Other narratives have lost their urgency. Other narratives have been lost altogether. No matter what we know, no matter what we hear at the TRC or find in the archives, there are always questions unasked and unanswered, things not told, motivations unspoken, placed unrecorded, graves unmarked or unmarkable.

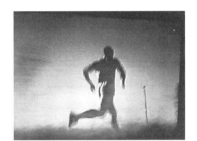

In the absence of tangible relics so much is invested in our gaze on the land. The act of looking and finding an image becomes the memorial or substitutes for it until another, more complete, can be made. We gaze at and probe the earth in the hope that we can discern in a wash of sand, a dispersed or chance pile of stones, mound, or hollow, some evidence that this might be the spot where a life ended, a dream was confirmed or lost. Land absorbs history and all but the grandest traces of action. In that sense, history is everywhere about us. Whilst the evidence of the moment is quickly lost, yet still the presence of place persists, and we construct from traces, however intangible. So what are we left with? . . . A sense that the air, a sighting of muddy river, or that outcrop of rock so implacably bland in the light of midday, is undertowed by memory. My attention is forever fluctuating between that which is known, the 'implacably bland', and the more insistent void of the fugitive.

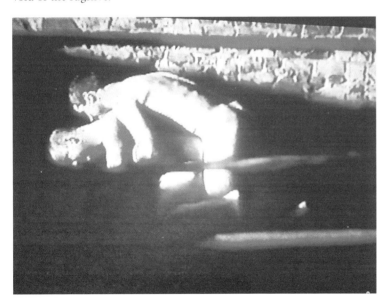

previous
underdelicacy

there

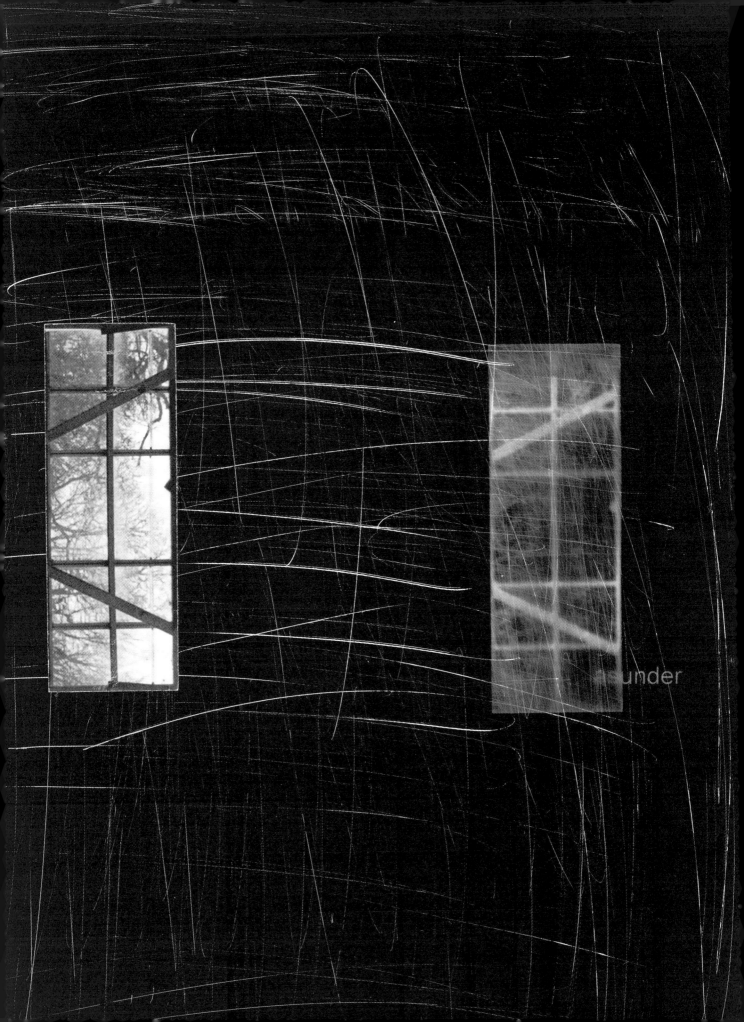

under

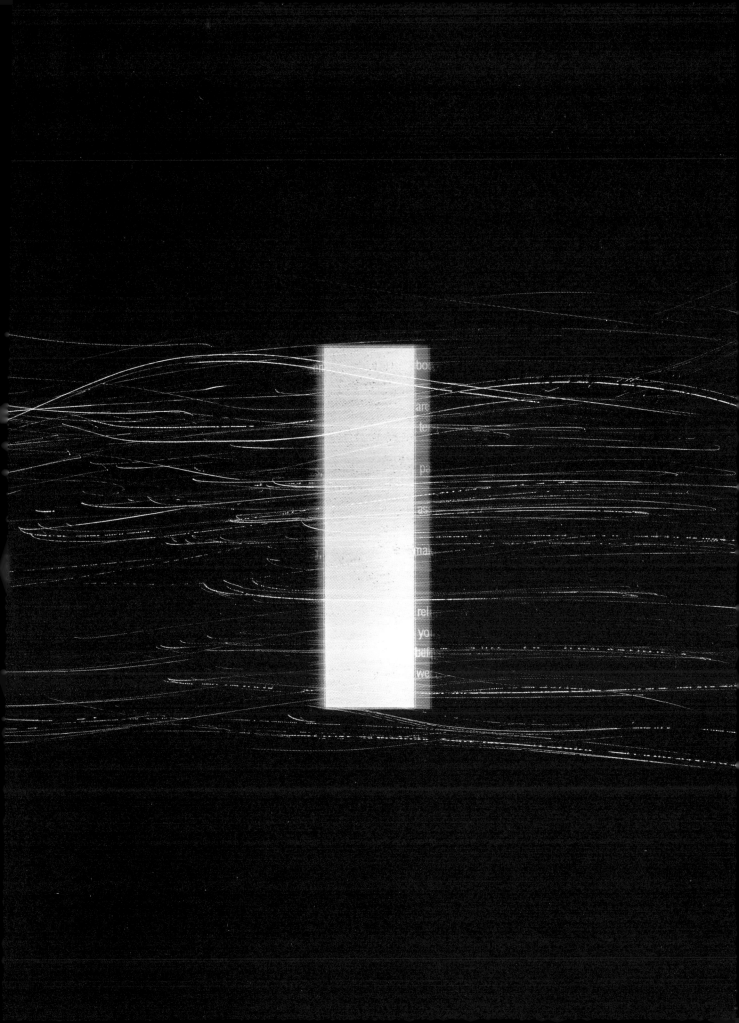

The Angel's Hideout:
Between Dance and Theatre

Enrique Pardo

Molti parlano di ispirazione di anima e nessuno di cultura.
Quando io parlo del corpo alludo alla cultura, perché la cultura è un corpo.
Se il cibo modella l'anima, la cultura modella i trati somatici,
rende viscerale o no il nostro sentire.*

Many speak of the soul's inspiration, no one of culture.
When I speak of body, I am referring to culture, because culture is a body.
If food shapes the soul, culture shapes the somatic traits,
makes our capacity to feel visceral or not.

* Alda Merini, in *La pazza della porta accanto* (Milan: Bompiani, 1995). In June 1996, I directed a choreographic theatre piece based on Merini's writings about her relationship with a tramp named Titano: 'Often while he made love to me, I was "elsewhere". My absence excited him because it is the way prostitutes offer themselves: smoking the cigarette of dreams.' The title of the piece was 'Mozzicone' – the polite Italian word for cigarette butts (Milan/Asti, 1996: an Estia, Buratto, Alfieri production). Merini's writings, and tragic life, are quite extraordinary; she was put forward for the Nobel Prize – it went to fellow Italian Dario Fo.

Our century has seen a succession of artistic expeditions towards a promised land somewhere between dance and theatre, a performance geography where literature and the physical body might meet, enhance each other's possibilities, and yield more complex images than they would if they were staged as protagonists in their own domain. This article is about one such expedition, a piece created in 1995/6 with five dancers; it addresses specific strategies of an approach to dance-theatre – I will tend to speak of *choreographic theatre* – and includes mythological reflections on dance as seen by an outsider. It also presents a militant view of emotion in performance, one that brings in angelology: the 'angels' hideout' as the possible place referred to by Alda Merini, where 'our capacity to feel visceral(ly) or not' is shaped, educated, per-formed: emotion as an '*ange qui dérange*', as a disturbing angel.

The search for dance-theatre hybrids gets attacked by purists on both sides. Official French theatre policy is designed to produce 'authors' (and hopefully, one day, France's much longed-for Shakespeare). The emphasis is fundamentally literary: theatre, as it will pass into history, is seen primarily on the printed page; words rule the stage, often in torrential deliveries. French dance milieux, on the other hand, and especially during the late 1980s, invoked the notion of *théâtralité* (theatrical-ity), usually defined as that which remains in theatre after words have been taken away. For many choreographers, this was an opening into a new semiotics of dance, a way out of the canons of strictly gestural composition. For the purists, it was gimmickry. From my point of view, if dance-theatre wishes to confront language, the spoken word, and connect to its metaphorical and emotional impli-cations, it cannot stop at movement with some

Performance Research 3(2), pp.19-26 © Routledge 1998

voice effects, or at the exploration of aleatoric juxtapositions of gesture and word.

My own artistic roots are a hybrid jumble, professionally (visual arts, voice performer, corporeal training, etc.) and culturally; but I am primarily concerned with language, the elaboration of metaphors that include the spoken word – and it is in the performing arts that I feel one can best 'realize', give body to the metaphorical, imaginal potential of language. I come from theatre (initially through voice work), and moved to contemporary dance (and corporeal mime, and other traditions) to find a working dialogue not only with eloquent and moving bodies, but with *choreography*: how choreography elaborates a 'con-text', a place, a landscape of relations and moves, a physical dramaturgy that can withstand the impact of 'text', and of the 'authoritarian' power of literature, and not be reduced to an illustrative frame.

DIALOGUES WITH DANCE

We inhabit and dance our bodies as mythical temples. There are many gods and goddesses, and each has his or her temples and rituals; each has his or her own 'theatre'. An archetypal approach to dance studies its images and principles in the very roots of culture, in the figures and stories of mythology. Placing dance in a polytheistic context of cultural diversity and of aesthetic differences encourages multiplicity (all mythic wars start with exclusions!), as well as critical confrontation.*

* From Pantheatre's 'choreographic theatre' yearly professional training program in France.

Before moving into specific strategies pertaining to the interplay between dance and theatre, some remarks on dance from an outsider's point of view, one searching for a choreographic collaboration.

1 Diana's Bath: Dance and Virginity

Contemporary dance studios are often temples of 'feeling', pervaded by a mystique of sensitivity. The mood in them can be quintessentially Artemisian (Artemis, the Roman Diana): private, feminine, soft, delicate, pure, devoted to febrile and

sometimes fanatical listening to *inner* sensations. The atmosphere is that of Diana at her bath: clear water and pristine wilderness, protected groves, untainted by any hint of specularity or seduction (except of course for the narcissism of mirrors when they appear – but that is another matter; here I am referring to the gaze of the spectator). The image of Diana and her nymphs washing their limbs offers a personified picture of nature's virginal ecology: no artifice, but devoted care for the 'right' postures and optimum muscle tone. Serious, sensitive, silent, usually pale, and tremendously self-involved. We are as far as can be from one of the original words for 'actor': *hypokritos*.

Karine Saporta, a leading and spectacular choreographer, something of France's contemporary Cleopatra, blasts at the precious privacy in these attitudes. Charismatic, fiery and bitingly eloquent, she is in turn reviled for breaking bodies and reducing them to puppets; her shows do not skirt *femme fatale* theatrics and luxurious pageants – she choreographed the dance for Peter Greenaway's *Prospero's Books*. She accuses Artemisian devotees of reaching degrees of sensitivity where they can no longer bear the gaze of a spectator – the ultimate withdrawal of dance from show.

This quarrel has mythical dimensions. The hunter Actaeon was torn to pieces by his own hounds for watching Artemis/Diana at her bath, for introducing an Aphroditean gaze into a virginal setting; Artemis would accuse him of pollution and pornography. Not only is there a sense in which one is not supposed to gaze at Artemisian moves, but, in their so-called natural, pure, even wild aesthetic, there is a refusal of metaphorical displacement; dance is a question of being, certainly not of showing, or of allowing an associative glance. If Artemis (personified in a woman or a man) passes your way, admire the transparent freshness of her/his swift body, fit and nimble, svelte and slender, the transfiguration of her/his healthy well-being. . . . Enjoy the shine, the athletic allure, the sporty companionship, the sibling enthusiasm she/he might share with you. But, if transparency is resented and you sense a refusal of your gaze and of your presence as a spectator, if there is a protective reaction of privacy (what has been called the goddess's 'vicious shyness'), then one is confronting a dangerous Artemis, one that must not be drawn into theatre but left to celebrate her private rituals. One also encounters, as in all closed mythological schools, something that could be called 'Artemisian proselytism': the righteousness of those who are not interested in your performance, but who want to put your bodies 'right'.

2 Aphrodite's Specularity

Diana's baths are very different from Aphrodite's (or Hera's), by which the goddess renews her virginity in order to reoffer it every night, afresh. Diana's bath takes place after the hunt – hunting being her preserve. There is symbiosis between the goddess and her animals: wild, fast, fresh, alert. Hunting for her is an athletic and exhilarating identification with the hunted. Artemisian abstraction (abstracted out of metaphor, among other things) partakes of these game patterns: the stage as a clearing traversed by fast, fleeting silhouettes, visited by diaphanous presences. Diana's identification with hunting involves killing; she both protects and hunts down her animals, tracking, outsmarting and finally surprising them for the kill. She is a detached killer, striking from a distance, with arrow or javelin, like her brother Apollo, and unlike Dionysus's maenads who tear animals (and children, and men . . .) with their bare hands and teeth. Diana's bathing comes after all the sweat, the running, the exacting and exhilarating competition, the keen adrenalin and its ultimate release in the kill. The bath is a private grooming, a proud and soothing reward to one's wild animal body, muscle tone and healthy skin, and to one's killing fitness. She is often pictured sharing this ritual with her shy and ferocious greyhounds.

Aphrodite, on the other hand, rejoices in looks. As *Porneia*, she embraces pornography within her domains of 'grace' – at war with current puritanism, which wants to get rid of its obscenity (socioeconomical, for instance) by unloading it on to pornography. Aphrodite blesses the intercourse between vision and sex, arouses the world through looks, disseminates beauty through specular desire, through display: cosmetics enhancing the cosmos. In the stories where she is betrayed, flouted or mocked, she is as murderous as Artemis, or any repressed goddess or god for that matter. Repressed principles return with a fanatical and tyrannical outlook, rejecting theological alternatives, let alone allowing any form of mythical democracy, and therefore refusing to enter into a theatre that would include but relativize their aesthetics.

3 Le Théâtre de la Ville

In the last fifteen years, contemporary French dance performances have been drawn into a vortex whose top model and ambition is Le Théâtre de la Ville, with its huge, frontal stage for some 2,000 spectators, akin to a steep movie house, or worse – and especially with dance – to a grand aquarium. The expectation is one of 'major' performances, and choreographers have stumbled willy-nilly into productions that last over an hour in order to fulfil this model. Rarely do they present, as in the past, a repertoire program of dance pieces. The Pina Bausch monumental model prevails over, say, a Merce Cunningham program. Very few performances can sustain their propositions beyond thirty minutes, if that, and one ends up with long 'assemblages', drawn-out variations on a particular theme or aesthetical atmosphere, or extended collages exploiting two or three basic choreographic or scenographic parameters. Rarely can one speak of them as having any sense of depth dramaturgy, mythical complexity, or psychological substance.

Choreography is one thing, tackling theatre models is another. French dance blossomed during the 1980s (*les années fric*), fearlessly using the 'major' model, and fully promoted by fashionable socialism (under Jack Lang's flashy reign as minister of culture). The contrast with Britain is worth observing, Britain being a poor relation as far as state subsidies to the arts are concerned. Attitudes there tend to be much tougher, with an avowed allergy to French 1980s' dance-theatre proposals. The most violent reactions came from two camps: the abstract-dance purists (who, to a large extent, perform by the frugal ethics of Artemis); and what I call the British Cromwellian tendency – punkish, anti-arty, aggressive, and, to a great extent, northern 'Protestant' iconoclasts. Their battle-cry belongs to yet another mythical (and historical) war, in this case a war against French 'Catholic', 'effeminate' cultural icons, and it can be a very refreshing and salutary reaction, salting and grounding artistic endeavour. But this particular kind of puritanical iconoclasm can also be regressively and tyrannically anti-cultural, and end up worshipping some dour, nihilistic and barbarian Saturn.

CHOREOGRAPHIC THEATRE

Two working principles: *Conversion* and *Contradiction*

No single label can do justice to the fullness or complexity of an artistic research. My own reason for preferring 'choreographic theatre' to other terms such as 'dance-theatre' or 'physical theatre' is because it contains chorus, graphics and theatre. It implies bodies in image, and the 'theatre' between them – which, again, includes the spoken word, language, text, as one of its fundamental components. The other components of image are: the visual (all *graphia*: gestural, choral, pictorial), language (literary images), the voice (which, like dance, can be separate from or even contradict language, and trigger its own realm of music and images), and music.

I wish to focus on two working principles particularly concerned with the dynamic between dance and language. The aim is to be able to move back and forth between dance and language, to alternate between the two, to juxtapose and intermingle them, and above all to metamorphose them into each other. The first principle is that of 'conversion' – conversion from dance to text, and back again. Conversion, first, as in religion, like St Paul, knocked off his high horse (and getting on to another one!) on the road to Damascus. This

implies the capacity to radically change one's driving faith, styles and systems of expression. It speaks for versatility and casuistics (an adult, adulterous and adulterating process), the capacity for alternation and change. Secondly, conversion as in thermodynamics, where heat is turned into movement and vice versa: waterfalls into electricity, fuels exploding into speed, or imploding into diamonds. Essential within this more mechanistic approach to conversion is the capacity to dissociate; like training to play the piano with two hands, one gains the artistic autonomy to join or separate language and gesture, including counterpoint, syncopation, dynamic transfers, and the musical control of emotion and energy (which tend to be primordial, organic, associative, 're-membering' factors).

Third, conversion as in the early days of psychiatry, where the 'syndrome of conversion' was played out in the great nineteenth-century amphitheatres, and key words yielded extraordinary feats of 'physical theatre': histrionics, *logos* spectacularly transformed into *soma*, psychosomatic drama, what came to be called hysteria. Much has been written about this 'theatre', whose benches laid the foundations for Freud's theories.* What interests me is not the theatrical setting, but the underlying principles: association/conversion, the 'transport' (*metaphorein*) from one realm to another, from language to body gestures and symptoms – poetry being an associative activity (at least as far as language is concerned). Here, the model implies that through conversion, psyche (the unconscious, memory, or imagination) is enacted and displayed in dance or, 'conversely', articulated in language. Meaning is extracted, shaped, converted back and forth between movement and language, each mutation a new commentary, a fresh layer of repercussions, a further poetical 'realization'. ('To realize

* The year 1996 marked the centenary of the founding of psychoanalysis. The theatrics of hysteria and of memory, so crucial to the birth of psychoanalysis, again made sensational headlines with the postponement of the planned Freud centenary exhibition at the Library of Congress, Washington DC. On hysteria, Sonu Shamdasani, one of the scholards who 'signed' the postponement petition, had this to say: 'I have always understood hysteria to be a hypnotic artefact invented by physicians and cloned by patients.'

what one is saying or doing' means to realize the 'metaphorical reality' of a gesture or an expression.)

'Realization' is at the core of the performer's craft; she/he is inside image, is part of it, 'realizing' its body, giving it metaphorical reality. Conversion is one of the main tools in this instinctual hermeneutics, in the craft of dramatic interpretation: the meanings that emerge from how, when, why one shifts from language to movement. It means *making significant moves* within image, listening and 'realizing' what the overall image is saying, how it is coming across to the spectators. These 'moves' enrich, complexify, deepen its metaphorical body (or blast it through an iconoclastic initiative). Developing *the instinct of image* – an animal sense of image that allows for instinctual conversion moves – is the main point of choreographic theatre training.

The second working principle is the notion of 'contradiction'. In theatre, language can be 'the enemy', usurping the body's autonomous expressivity, subduing dance, for instance, into a secondary illustrative or decorative mode. Textual dictatorship can impose its authoritarian grip through so-called respect for the author, or through traditions of interpretation that constrain performing artists into set and often stale cultural moulds. Its tyranny on fiction can lead to rhetorical sclerosis, to linear story-telling and declamatory clichés. In training, at least, I treat texts as enemies, paying them a higher tribute, and giving interpreters a chance to live up to them, to face up to them. The strategy is one of *contra-diction* (against-diction) and *inter-diction*: inhibiting and making the delivery of words a prohibiting affair, coming under an interdict, repressing, arresting any naive approach to speech. This might sound forbidding, but the aim is actually to deliver the performer from the tyrannical power of language – an inevitable outcome if one goes to texts as Red Riding Hood went to the woods: the wolf of literature will get you. Resistance gives body to text (more on this below). I encourage '*negative listening*': the capacity both to listen to and to resist the text, even to counter it. This strategy is close to

Keats's notion of 'negative capability': the ability to hold one's place as a performer when faced with the poetic polysemy of image, not to rush to an interpretation and allow complexity to proliferate.

The notion of contradiction differs from modernistic aleatoric performance procedures, where, for instance, a recorded speech is switched on, preferably of neutral delivery, while the performers count their steps in a dance routine, without connection, without emotion, without resistance – 'deadpan' encounters in a universe ruled by cool (and sometimes frozen) Kronos-like principles of geometric chance.*

* The differentiation between aleatoric and spontaneous outlooks, and the mantic and serendipitous traffic between them, is at the core of patterns of inspiration, and of age-old mythical wars: for instance, the one between abstraction and figuration. In his 'Pan and the Nightmare' (CT: Spring Publications, 1972), James Hillman tackles this area from the god Pan's perspective, and the principle of panic. Pantheatre was named in part after this essay.

CHOREOGRAPHIC THEATRE: THE SEX OF ANGELS

Choreography, from this particular bias, is a mythography of sorts; it writes and reads patterns of relationships in a figurative cosmology. It transforms abstract space into places, revealing the potential exchanges between characters within mythological dramaturgies, and exploding, like dance, one-dimensional naturalism. It lets imagination breed in the angelic interstices; it gives density to the air through personifications, it constellates presences in-between realities. Before releasing language into choreographic image-making, and in order to withstand its impact, choreography must first consolidate its own *con-text*: its own web of relations, stories, identities. When this con-text is solid enough, one can bring in text, so that text and context can meet, clash, dance, and this with full paradoxical impact.

A striking psychological definition of body once put forward by James Hillman in the context of theatre was that there is body wherever there is *resistance*. With provocative conciseness, and elegance, it sums up Psyche's perspective on body, caught in the double bind of desire and resistance of her relationship with Eros: his need for blind erotic involvement, hers for enlightenment – the need to confront the object of her desire. The physical bliss of her nights with Eros is sheer literal body; the suffering after the separation gives her metaphorical body – she breaks sexual fusion by lighting the candle and 'realizing' who her lover really is. (She also creates 'confusion', another important choreographic principle!)*

* See Apuleius's story of Psyche and Eros.

Each school of thought lives its ideas of what body is as an ontological experience, and we all risk being fundamentalist about it. The idea that gives body to that so-called 'ontological experience' is much more difficult to apprehend since it surrounds and defines our very sense of being, and its ways of experiencing; it shapes our aesthetics, our modes of perception, and our evaluation of that perception. '*Notre méconnaissance forme un système fermé, rien ne peut la réfuter*' ('Our ignorance constitutes a closed circuit, nothing can refute it': Christa Wolf, in *Medea*, 1996). It takes substantial cultural reflection to identify the idea that is moving us, and that 'salts' our experience and its pleasures.

I tend to place my working definition of body in territories similar to Hillman's. It is a semantic approach that finds body every time it encounters *the angel of meaning*: making sense, sensual meaning. There is body when associations coagulate; when persons, objects and the air around them are visited and animated by presences, memories, spirits – epiphanies, manifestations; when metaphors rise, run and rain – body as sustained revelation, giving 'body' to our own physical bodies . . . matter awakened, quickened, set into motion by ideas . . . meaning as movement, movement as meaning . . . metamorphoses . . . objects, muscles, bones, skin, alive, transmuted, inhabited, moved . . . metaphoric animals, angels, and the flow of understandings . . . realizations, poetical harvests . . .

Underlying such a litany, especially one invoking angelology, is a basic philosophical bias; it requires the move from motion to emotion, and it says that

there is body wherever there is emotion. The encounter with the angel of meaning is permeated with emotion; ideas come enfolded in its wings. But the poor word (emotion) is so tired of being measured and calibrated in pharmacology, of being whipped up and acted out in all sorts of therapies, that one hardly dares to use it any more. To give emotion back some mythological life I would propose that what we call emotions today were once called angels – acknowledging that this is an overtly militant, mytho-poetical move. First, it removes emotion from personal, subjective ownership; rather than being 'ours' or 'in us', emotions possess us. Inspiring presences, visitations, personified powers, emotions move us, often overwhelming, sometimes crushing – divine influxes, messengers from the ruling or unruly gods. They come with divine intention, and power, and handle the synapses between message and biology, mind and adrenalin. They 'make' sense, at once intellectual and emotional. If there is no angel, there is 'no-body'.

The Greek *angelos* means 'messenger', and the arch-messenger in Greek mythology is Hermes, a god too often and too conveniently reduced to cybernetics, or at best to an ambivalent communications principle. To rehabilitate angelology, especially a 'hermetic' one, and to shake off its aura of cute religiosity, we should return to the pagan figure of *daimon*, which holds together good angel, nasty demon and a lot more.[†] Fra Angelico's brigades of winged youths, all the same in neat uniforms, in fanatical ranks singing up to 'the one and only' god, can be seen as pious antecedents of not-so-distant parades on the Red Square, or, worse, at Nuremberg, sprinkled with gold and artificial snow . . . Hermes was anything but sexless and neutral. The Homeric Hymn is explicit: he spends most of

[†] Recent scholarship has revisited the notion of emotion as daimonic, enlarging considerably the blinkers of scientist and anthropological thinking. See especially Ruth Padel, *In and Out of the Mind: Greek Images of the Tragic Self* (Princeton, NJ: Princeton University Press, 1992); and *Whom Gods Destroy: Elements of Greek and Tragic Madness* (Princeton, NJ: Princeton University Press, 1995). For a mind-opening reactualization of the notion of daimon, placed at the core of personality, see James Hillman, *The Soul's Code* (New York: Random House, 1996).

his time making love with nymphs in soft, dark, moss-covered caverns. Read it this way: the 'principle of communication', so-called neutral, is intimately, sexually and constantly involved with nymphs, with alluring anima figures, with the driving fantasies of life, with the feminine personifications of the world.

LA PLANQUE AUX ANGES

The Angels' Hideout (*La Planque aux Anges*) is a shady, canal-side 'cruising' area in downtown Strasbourg, hosting a succession of dubious activities, mainly to do with sex and drugs, as described by the French playwright Bernard Marie Koltès in an early novel of his, *La fuite à cheval/très loin dans la ville* (The Horseback Flight Far into Town); I adapted the novel as a performance in 1995–6. Koltès is probably the most performed playwright in France today; his plays involve drop-out characters spinning webs of words around each other, in a unique mixture of seductive argumentation, aggressive zaniness and disarming lyricism. These plays are also overwhelmingly literary – avalanches of words.

In adapting this novel, we skirted the tidal wave of his language, and the often heavy dialectical architecture. One critic described *La Planque aux Anges* in terms of cinema: images, actions and the minimum of necessary dialogues, no tirades, no spoken metaphysics – barely five pages of text. This piece was performed by five dancers, some of whom had practically no experience of spoken theatre. They trained in a two-year research program called *Borderline*, exploring the frontiers of dance-theatre, and venturing into borderline deconstructions of images and characters. All five performers were 29 or 30 years old, having trained and worked with major, and quite disparate, French and American dance companies. We chose Koltès together; paradoxically the play's characters are mostly younger in age than the performers, but so scorched, hurt, lived, that their despair, and soul's age, seemed often out of reach.

La Planque aux Anges took off as a radical venture, with few concessions, and it was surprising

to see, on arrival, the kind of acting that emerged, and how it flowed into dance or out of it. The association with cinema initially surprised me, but made strong sense; all five dancers had accepted an adventure into highly strung acting, the stuff most of us in theatre (and so much more so in dance) have relinquished to film, with its close-ups on 'realistic' emotional acting. Usually, when tears appear on stage I fear the worst: being dragged through thick tragedies and hours of overacting – emotions stylized into literary monuments. Yet it is something that in movies seems lighter and acceptable; to a large extent, realistic emotional acting, the legendary stuff of the Actors' Studio, has been handed over to films and TV. *La Planque aux Anges* rebelled against this so-called give-away, wishing to retrieve the stuff of emotions back to live, dancing bodies, without getting caught in ceremonial drama, and without bowing to the hypnotic paradise of movies, much as I enjoy it. As far as I am concerned, nothing can replace the challenge of a live performance, providing one can touch and be touched by its mythical pulse, brushed by its 'wings of desire'.

In retrospect, it can be said that the piece 'zoomed' in on emotions as they rose from contradictions, and 'panned' after their conversions. Spectators sat at the edge of both sides of a long, narrow performing area (12 x 5 metres), divided into three sections, or 'rooms': they were placed where the walls of the flat would have been, and confronted only one of the three rooms, with a partial view of the other two. No one had a detached, overall view – not only was the spectator not in a position of visual overlord, but he/she felt something of an intruder into the characters' lives and space. A voyeur, peering into a hideout where angels were at work, distilling emotions into dance, or cornering it into some form of singing. Sometimes they (the hidden angels) made the characters go wild with shouting and dancing, or break down and cry alone in front of a mirror; sometimes they would lie in bed with them, idly dreaming in front of a TV screen, occasionally gathering these strands into one of Koltès's speeches.

The program dedicated the piece to 'the children of Hecate', drop-outs who loiter in nocturnal gangs with the bag-lady goddess and her stray dogs, rummaging society's wastebins at the 'trivia', the crossroads at the city outskirts. These are society's 'refuse', said to be the unsettled souls of violent and asocial deaths: victims of overdoses, murders, suicides, car crashes. They are the interfering, marauding spirits of occultism: spiritual pollution. *La Planque aux Anges* was presented during the August 1995 'Myth and Theatre' festival dedicated to 'Magic', and it shocked those who came to the festival with salvationist expectations (magic as hope), or sensationalist ones (magic as shamanic surrealism). Although the piece made no overt reference to mythology (or to magic, for that matter), it invited in some of their darker angels. These stirred the air, upset and blew the characters' moods about. One did not confront grand allegories, black or white magic, but an in-between, borderline, complex world made of contradictions, trivia, shadows, unhappy characters – insecure figures adrift, yet managing to hold on to rare and precious moments of humour, tenderness, poetry and dance. They danced against all odds: physical and psychological. The setting was claustrophobic, crowded and cluttered; dancing was hard earned and rose out of emotionally loaded texts and contexts, a density that, hopefully, gave the performers and their dance the sort of 'body' I have tried to describe here.

Little Tyrannies, Bigger Lies:

a Letter from the Other Side

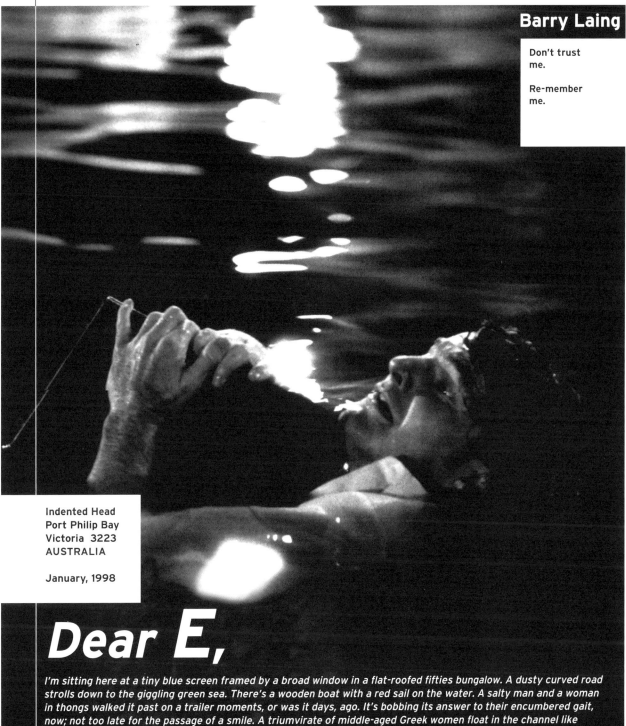

Barry Laing

Don't trust
me.

Re-member
me.

Indented Head
Port Philip Bay
Victoria 3223
AUSTRALIA

January, 1998

Dear E,

I'm sitting here at a tiny blue screen framed by a broad window in a flat-roofed fifties bungalow. A dusty curved road strolls down to the giggling green sea. There's a wooden boat with a red sail on the water. A salty man and a woman in thongs walked it past on a trailer moments, or was it days, ago. It's bobbing its answer to their encumbered gait, now; not too late for the passage of a smile. A triumvirate of middle-aged Greek women float in the channel like cloves of garlic cackling oily Christmas tales between swells. Caravans huddle together in the park on the foreshore. A pelican on the bridge of a tanker steers the hulk through the heads, its own wings too soon less sure of flight. There are whale bones on the beach; ribs, a wreck of breath, splitting the breeze with howling, pushing, breaking the waves. A boat. My heart. This cage ... of memory where the whale has swum, and me in the belly of the whale – unseeing, unknowing – and yet I swim: memory in me treading water; beached, bleached like a daguerreotype.

Hello. I'm hoping you may re-member me – I went missing, dis-appeared, for a while – from a series of encounters in 1993 and 1994. London, Paris, the south of France. You introduced me to Philippe Gaulier, Monika Pagneux, Théatre de Complicité, Pantheatre and Anzu Furukawa. You spoke, whispered to me, casually. I found myself asking the 'Does a Little Tyranny need a Bigger Lie' question – whining sometimes, persistent – but not before you suggested, heuristically, cumulatively, that 'Lies' might be understood as critical fictions, illusion, artifice, transgression, pretence, pretension, insolence, stupidity, and re-presentations: contrary, for example, to the 'Little Tyranny' of capital T 'Truth' and capital E 'Emotion' in certain kinds of theatre, dance and psychological discourse. You sung of discursive tyrannies – capital R 'Real' in performance – but unilaterally, depending on the angle of vision or the 'place' from which one looks, 'tyrannies' of all kinds: 'musical' tyrannies, spatial ones, political correctness, habitude, prostheses, 'hip', Democracy, Physical Theatre even, diplomacy, the words 'I love you', politeness, surface, psychological depth, and anxiety. [*The whale belches the vagaries of Hijikata's claim that anxiety is like the kid who pisses his pants before the race has begun ...*]

I was a tourist. Now I am a missive ...

There was a stampede in heaven – or was it Hades – and the sixteen hooves of the horses of the horsemen of an apocalypse, a domestic one, weak, and sad, in a tiny room with a pane onto a grey wall ... these sixteen hooves I met with my four, in time. Call them; Love, Faith, Honour, Forgiveness. My four hooves, and me my only defender; and the only betrayal my own if I fail to meet the others at the gates of my heart. To turn them away. And I am the Unicorn. You are here inside the walls – not out there where night approaches – cracking fire, flintstone under foot. Me my defender. You my heart. The night ablaze all around. Me my defender. You my heart. As the flickering shadows keep time with destruction. Me my defender. You my heart. And Grace between us. Grace.

Love. Faith. Honour. Forgiveness. You inside the walls? Here? Already here? Awake. It is the sweet smell of me feathered and ghosted on your thighs. I will visit you there, again and again, sleeping safe in my heart.

Gaulier grumbled, 'You can't cheat with your humanity'. It is a question of liberty: we glimpsed it as freedom with limits. I say 'we', but I'm covering for you.

Terra Incognita - land unknown.
Terra *Nullius* - empty land.
Terra Australis.

Poems on a Melbourne Tram, 1995

'Dreaming place ...
You can't change it.
No matter you rich man,
No matter you king.
You can't change it.'

Bill Niedge

'More than repair,
everything is in
need of mercy ... .'

Peter Bukowski

Dear B,
To travel from Australia to Europe full of the illusions and critical fictions of the wilful force of a desire which would announce Europe as *the* site of learning and inquiry whiffs of a very familiar 'Cultural Cringe'. Where's your culture? *E*

[*In sepia tones I remember how in Western Australia in 1990 I learned that South African Nationalists sent a working party to WA in 1947 to study state legislation. They borrowed half a dozen or so of our laws enacting the good-will of a white supremacist Australia and promptly returned to include them in draft legislation for an Apartheid South African State in 1948. Apartheid's 'un-Australian'. We wave the flag for sanctions. But don't trust me. I'm a liar.*]

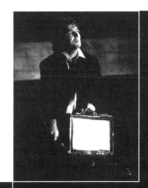

... I have a vision! I see a City: tall buildings, lights on every street corner – bright lights – towers and beacons, pathways and factories. Billowing smoke. Industry. Coal and iron and steel. *Prodigious machinery* ... Yes, we'll build a city ... here! ... But, there are natives in the bushes, eyes peering from the darkness, all around, sniggering, playing didgeridoos! You! – scout around in front, I'll come up behind. Round them up. *Drive them into the river!!!* The river ... ahhh, there, at the bend, we'll build a Great City ... and for you, a white house, with white, carved posts at the verandah overlooking the water. And there, a blue boat tied with a rope to a jetty. A bright blue boat, tugging at its rope ... here at the bend ... *drive them into the river!!!* ... We'll build a city, a Great Nation and ... Oh, *yes*, there'll be joy and laughter like a babbling brook. You, take the oars. I'll stand at the prow. We'll course this great river ... row on, I say, onward! Here a mill, there a store-house. Row on ... love your work!

I'm a yes-sayer. Positive. Never said no in my life except to say, 'Yes. No, *really* – I love your work'. I'm positive. I'm HIV positive. Trust me.

Dearest *E*,
You have taken me from this 'site' – my experience of Australia – to London, Paris and back again. There is in this movement a 'circle', a collocatory set of encounters in ignorance, inspiration [*the whale breathes in*], revelation, and insights ruptured by time and questioning place. I am in-formed by this circle. The circle is de-scribed by me, inscribed in me. The question of 'place', the site from which one looks, sees or enquires and the site/s by and via which the travelling 'Self' is interrogated in turn, is enacted in the pedagogy and dramaturgy that flow from this experience – and this writing which constitutes part of its praxis.

'Selves' conspire - *multiple*. The world dances, turns. There is movement. Monika Pagneux sang, 'Everything is music'. I believed her. Gaulier complained, 'Belief is not necessary. Believe nothing.'

In the studio we've been walking, walking, walking. Breaking up the 'I' that walks.

[*A tale breaks the surface, the bulb flashes. Burns. Smoke clears revealing a murder of crows throat singing in protest on the opposite shore ... Llllllllrrrrrraaaaaaaaaaaarrrrrrrrrrrrrrrrrrk ...*

... Ohhhhhh, I have memories of the CIRCUS! where, rushed by a clown with a bucket full of water, I fell through the wooden seating in terror only to open my eyes to spiralling confetti in colours I had not yet imagined. I remember the rhythms of work and the smell of my leather satchel, and I remember play, and the words of poets sent from lovers before they ever loved me. I remember – when the opaque winds come swirling in – I remember a place with a heart. People, and images, and words that were blessings ...]

E, you were already here. I've been trying to 'take place', 'make an appearance': conjuring concepts of 'Presence' and its shadow, 'Absence' – positions mirrored in the Occidental/Oriental divide. I've been marking marginalities, plotting peripheries and diagnosing dis-appearances as if you were elsewhere. As if you were other.

The eulogy of 'The Other'. The Return of the Same.

[*Flash. I strike a match in the putrid darkness. Flames – initiation by fire. Understanding comes.*]

I attempt to draw the other towards me, all the while holding firm in my own contradictory discourse of 'opening', and yet not knowing really what it is to stand in relationship with another;[1] to love, to be in love. I've been waiting for you, as if when you arrived, so would I. But I've been waiting for 'me' – and I simply haven't known what would shake the foundations of my solitude, the fixed, lonely foot in me: the clenched jaw, the tight chest – the 'mask' with which I have divided myself. Ohhh, I've been crying and crying and crying as if to give voice to my pain would somehow bring compassion down upon me. From where, I don't know ... More than repair everything is in need of mercy. But you are here, already here.
Melbourne, Victoria, AUSTRALIA.

Dear B,
I've seen you walking in a landscape with tears. *Anzu*

Burn this page

18 May 1996

Dear RD,
I'm angry. Full of rage. I want to scream into the empty space.

[*In the darkness we roll against a swell and I hear thunder. It is the feet of the son of the father on the open stage of the Palais Royale in Paris. It's very hot. July, 1994. Kazuo Ohno teeters – funny, pathetic. But there is terror in a smile, and the imaginal skies threaten retribution. He is danced by an extraordinary fragility, and the simultaneous presence of a very young woman and the love of an old man: the span of a life in a gesture of yearning; an endless moment of loss. He speaks to me. I have forgotten when and from where. I hear his voice like a wind blowing, everything is music: 'I discovered I could dance when I learned that the space is not empty.'*]

We turn away, risking melanoma, sun on our backs.
'Outback', the interior.
We turn away.

The reality and the metaphor of 'The Desert' in your words is potent: the immensity of the place, the site itself; the 'desert' in others, in oneself; the struggle between 'Selves'; aloneness, loneliness; 'homelessness' (or 'home', for those not passing through); the imperishable place of 'memory'; independence; the potential desolation of the mind in 'time'; the 'glue' of the ego; and the sometimes terrible white-noise of rage. I have thought a lot about this 'rage' in me – in extremes while in India in 1989, while travelling up through the centre from Melbourne to Darwin, and in my weaker moments – as my 'Self' against all 'Others'.

James Hillman is a lion roaring. It's a question of the 'anaesthetized heart':

> What is passive, immobile asleep in the heart creates a desert. ... The more our desert the more we must rage, which rage is love. The passions of the soul make the desert habitable. ... The desert is not (outback); it is anywhere once we desert the heart. (Hillman in Moore 1990)

On a trip last year up through the Red Centre – Uluru, the Olgas, Alice, then Darwin – pretty much on the highway and only touching the edges of the 'real' desert, I became palpably aware of the desert I had swirling around my mind-wheels, encroaching on my soft, hidden, sleeping heart. The road sent my own 'music' back to me which was tricky at times and, it seemed, at every oasis or plunge-pool of my imagination there lurked the crocodile to death-roll the little ego; questioning my desires, dragging me out of complacencies, demanding that I deal with all I encountered on its own terms. I 'taught' performance in some schools and communities for Aboriginal kids on the way – just levelled me. Found myself dancing in a 'schoolyard' as the moon came up over the desert, music blaring, playing soccer and frisbee – simultaneously – and sharing a kind of intimacy and understanding that's defined by what's gone before here, wrongly, and by the 'chance' of us finding a way through it.

There were mornings of 'teaching' more than seventy 'kids' – some as young as 6, some initiated men, women who couldn't hold my gaze or do certain things in front of the men, and where anyway 'performance' for some was a 'shame job'. They taught me what can't be learned about what's going on out there from the sanitized and expertly counter-politicized place of these cities here, which hug the coastline as if it was their own 'hearts' they're most afraid of. But as Hillman wails, defying the infarct, the desert is not heartless because the desert is where the lion lives, and the lion sleeps in our heart, and we in the heart of the lion:

> Our way through the desert of life or any moment in life is the awakening to it as a desert, the awakening of the beast, that vigil of desire, its greedy paw, hot and sleepless as the sun, fulminating as sulphur, setting the soul on fire ... (ibid.)

On the flip-side of desire lurks the shadow of the 'Self', and accompanying rage is the possibility of silence. There's a kind of crippling silence of the heart which comes of excessive noise, but there's another kind of silence where time seems to spread out like a fan, spinning on itself, and where we don't measure its passing in violence to ourselves or others, or fill the present with the collisions of the shadows of future hopes and past sorrows. But the 'Self' will often have it another way.

In the studio we've been falling down. Falling to 'defy gravity'; greeting the lion's breath, and the howl of the world.

During a rare pause in the mad rage, frustration, and anger I found propelling me around India in 1989 – failing dismally at pretending not to be a tourist on my first trip anywhere – more rage! – I sat mesmerized by a huge crow on the window sill of an India Coffee House ...
[*There is a flurry of ragged wings and the glint of a sharp morning sun on angry bloody feathers. He's hanging there. Waiting. Beating in slow-motion against the sky. Just dis-appeared ...]*

REFERENCES:
Barthes, Roland (1990) *A Lover's Discourse*, Harmondsworth Mx: Penguin, Bly, Robert (1994) 'November Day at McClure's Beach', in *What Have I Ever Lost by Dying*, London: Weatherlight Press, Moore, Thomas (ed.) (1990) *The Essential James Hillman: A Blue Fire*, London: Routledge, Rose, Gilian (1995) *Love's Work: A Reckoning with Life*, New York: Schocken Books.
Sections of this text come from Barry Laing's solo performance, *Rapture* (La Mama, Melbourne, 1997).

... On a farm near a little town called Denmark in Western Australia. I'd been sent out, aged 11 or 12, to shoot crows that were threatening and killing newborn lambs. Squeeze, don't pull. Good shot. I lined up a bird in a tree, closed my eyes, squeezed – hoping I'd miss. The bird leaped from the branch, and flew ... and in that long silence after the explosion was a moment when I came close to vicarious flight. Hope, relief and all of life in an instant – but the wings of the bird buckled. I caught a single black feather between my fingers as it fell ...

Sometimes I see that bird, hanging there, hovering, except behind my eyelids now –
UNWANTED ANIMAL OCCUPANCY!

From where I sit, I can see in all its pallid hope a life that was never quite my own ... but I have glimpsed another world, and I have not yet come to terms with my grief.

... STOP THE FLUTTERING, STOP THE FLICKERING LIGHT ...

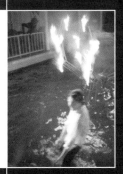

This 'grief' has been the shape of my experience sometimes, ahead of time. In my rage, and struggle to be in life, to 'take place', against fear, there is something of this kind of 'death' and 'dis-appearance' in the equation. But if such grief is part of the bargain, it augurs an insight of another kind:

> It is not our life we need to weep for. Inside us there is some secret. We are following a narrow ledge around a mountain, we are sailing on skeletal eerie craft over the buoyant ocean. (Bly 1994: 3)

Best wishes, B

As the great sherpa Philippe Gaulier once said to me at the foot of the mountain, "If you're heavy, just ... you die!".

No one ever drops in. I've done this all wrong.

I have *already* died, *already* lost love, *already* been abandoned, *already* felt the pain of annihilation, *already* forgotten my own dreamings, *already* suppressed my cry in the repression of the very moment I begin to take place – to live.

[*The receiver dangles on a taut cord in a phone box in Avignon, June 1993. The dial-tone follows me now into the belly of the whale, amplifies, transforms itself: it is the sound of the distended wingbeats of the crow, now the blades of a police helicopter in slow-motion overhead. And now, it is the voice of an old man who has loved – gravelly, dissident, calm: 'I am nowhere gathered together ... but I would burn rather than last'* (Barthes 1990: 11)]

Oh *E*, I digress. Unravelling the knots of disaffection in me: subjecting myself to muddles of multiplicity, cartographies of possible selves, geographies of possible sites; not trapped in a naturalist fallacy, 'caught' by a singular text, or lost in little tyrannies of any kind. You snatched me from a foreign shore, carried me away. *Rapture. Abduction. Transportation.* And in the circle of my 'return' there is the question of subjectification – how one might 'act' to convulse the imaginal field we inhabit, sometimes congregated too close to the centre where there's little room to move, even less for critical distance, and where life is stifled.

I was a tourist. Now I'm a missive ...

Re-member me.

B

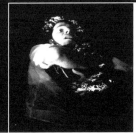

Dance Travels

Karen Pearlman

Dance travels.
Or does it?

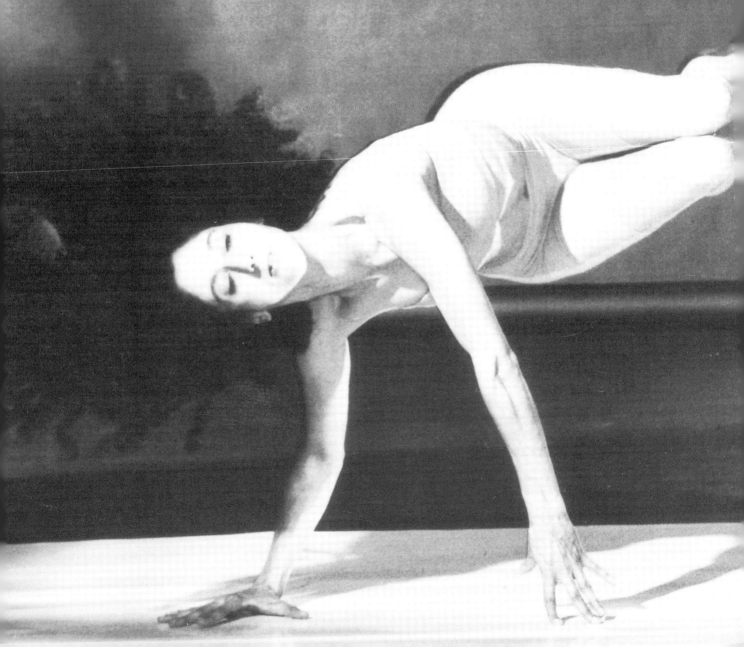

Start in the attic in Boston in 1964, waving scarves like Isadora, before going out to wave placards against the war. Dancing. At age 4.

St Louis, next, a site-specific work for the climbing frame in Flynn (named for Erroll) Park School playground. *Monkey Bar Blues* for five teenage girls dancing where they used to smoke but not inhale. Does the mark on the wall where we tried to set the building on fire five years earlier affect our current practice here? Or did the brick walls win, making us create structure in dance instead of havoc in the streets?

On the way to New York City (my spiritual home from the age of 12 when I began reading Deborah Jowitt in the *Village Voice*) I stop in North Carolina to see the world from everyone else's point of view. The American Dance Festival imports practice from all over the place to create a cafeteria-style dance world. I pig out, munching down jazzstyles from the cakewalk to the Lindy, anatomy from cerebellum to metatarsals, and latter-day Merce-enaries making a living by teaching chance.

Entranced by East Village sirens, I sign up for three years' hard labor at New York University, in whose converted ballrooms I pace, late, every Saturday night, looking for my original impulse and respite from the increasingly insistent chatter of inscriptions. The academy tries to pin down dance for us to learn it, but the too light fabric of the art form keeps shredding under the different dogma nails, leaving us in line and well aligned, but none the wiser.

Finally out and all alone I start the life I've been imagining myself made for for ten years. Being a glamorous dancer, meaning: sharing a sixth-floor walk-up in a battered tenement with Heywood McGriff, a hero among dancers and also broke; whizzing around the dingy downtown lofts at low rent hours; creating complex manipulations of movement material; sneakers; a shoulder bag; a bicycle; a waitressing job; a sense of purpose that went beyond job to be cause. I had it all. I even used to wait on Jim Jarmusch and John Lurie at

103 Second Avenue, but Paloma Picasso sat at someone else's table.

Timothy Buckley picked me out, after a six-month audition, to join his convoluted group of roustabouts, in *Out of the Blue*, *Barn Fever*, and *How to Swing a Dog*, four square, third generation Tharp, no two movements repeated, singular vision dances made in the right place at the right time to take us swinging around the grooviest of the dance places on the fringes of high culture and sometimes the middle of nowhere. Dancing Dusseldorf, White Plains, and West 19th Street with a kind of pre-grunge postmodernism that was generated by Timothy's transplant from the Ohio cornfields to the next wave catchers' field of New York in the early 1980s.

After our three years of near starvation on the totally cool but not quite ready for prime time circuit, the other three company members started having families or moving to Chicago, while I moved on to the Bill T. Jones/Arnie Zane Company. Here was a new place. A violent, heightened, fraught, incisive, aggressive, joy ride. The first place I'd been where what it looked like was more important than how it felt. A ground for shifting definitions of gender, strength, expression, style, personal politics, garments, the company you keep. Shifting them way out left, slingshotting them back to the right and up over the top, splatting into the face attached to the hand which fed us, and redirecting the mainstream by breaking down the back door with movement like machetes.

Leaving there to create my own place, I dropped the style thing, opting for my earlier grunge influences, but kept the guerrilla tactics. Partner/poet/Australian/dancer Richard James Allen and I formed That Was Fast, a company that could go anyplace, anytime, with dances in our pockets. Making a practice of never saying no, we danced in Manhattan from as far north as the 92nd Street Y to as far south as the Staten Island Ferry and in almost every outpost of postmodern dance in between. We saw almost every Pizza Hut salad bar in Britain on a tour of twenty-one cities, and almost as many train stations in Holland.

Karen Pearlman. Photo: Chris Callis

Stepping off the train in Portsmouth after Glasgow, Stirling, Shrewsbury, Sheffield, York, Cardiff, London, etc. – or, was it getting off the plane in Cincinnati after Adelaide, Melbourne, Canberra, Wollongong, Sydney, Townsville, Kuranda, Cairns – we suddenly realized that Mel Gibson had got there before us. Again. On the big screen. In *Lethal Weapon*. He'd been everywhere we'd been and more, and he personally hadn't moved. We began to shift the location of our practice from empty spaces, three-dimensionally present, to screens, wide or square, black and white or colour, but almost anywhere, even if always flat.

TV dance. We found conditions conducive to making it in Australia and so we shifted our company over here, and began transitioning between countries and their cultures, between spaces and their cultures. Dance, I found, is not a universal language if you are an ex-patriate trying to translate your native tongue. American dance is as different and same to Australian dance as America is to Australia. The cultural hegemonies are at once adored and despised, appreciated and resented, assimilated and perverted. I swim around, a fish out of context with a chip on my shoulder the size of my history, amazed at how little room to move there is in this huge expanse of space, and at the same time enjoying having my own cultural assumptions splintered into disposable pieces.

We try Tasmania, as artistic directors of Tasdance, where the price of access to screen facilities for making dance-that-can-go-anywhere is that we have to stay in Launceston, stewards of a fixed cultural institution. While there we also make several seriously mixed media shows, schools shows, the inaugural (and still active) Tasmanian Poetry and Dance Festival, and a new structure encompassing production in film, video, radio, publication and performance to try to update the notion of 'dance company' to something viable in the information age.

Maybe dance would be more universal if we didn't learn how to make it inside such culturally specific contexts. But everything, from what I thought one could say in dance to what I thought

one could wear while dancing, that was learned in New York was wrong in Tasmania. To my culturally inbred way of thinking you can only 'talk' in dance about things that can be expressed physically. So, sexual politics, for example, are a good subject for dance. Teapots, in my estimation, are not. Someone (a Tasmanian with influence and a real concern for the company) actually suggested we make dances about teapots. This was ironic because we had always used the teapot as an icon, a funny one, representing things that aren't really danceable. I didn't know where to begin to talk about what was obviously meaning-laden and metaphorically rich in the culture of people in Tasmania – the teapot. Not even a little one, short, stout or otherwise.

The places where contemporary dance is made and performed in New York are rough, dirty, ill-lit loft spaces in rough, dirty, ill-lit streets. But in Tasmania, our studios and theatres were polished, clean and well lit. And it seems our dance audiences were seeing the wrong reflection of place in our dances. It surprises me, after the Tasmanian experience, to come across comments, in the national newspaper, for example, about dance being a universal language. Perhaps it's wishful thinking, a huge, generative, underlying condition of humans to wish to be understood which makes us hope that even in our travels we can talk.

Back in Sydney now, the comparatively bustling metropolis, where we go next is as clear as it ever was and never is. But we practise everywhere we go, the places run off us leaving gullies and riverbeds marking places in our practice.

The art form is never staying in one place.

My Balls/Your Chin*

Mike Pearson

I want to tell you about Antonin Artaud and me.

I want to tell you about the work of RAT Theatre with whom I performed in 1972 and 1973. Of whom the programme for the Festival Mondial du Théâtre in Nancy said, 'few could, like them, legitimately, lay claim to Artaud, at least with regard to the manifesto on cruelty' and of whom Dutch newspaper *Het Parool* said, 'It is "Poor Theatre" and "Theatre of Cruelty" taken to their furthest extremes'.

* 'My Balls/Your Chin' is a piece by Last Exit from *Best of Live* (Enemy Records EMCD 110 1990).

If you look closely you can still see the stitch marks. Pounding a wooden crutch on the floor, it flew from my hand and hit me in the eye. Spent the rest of the performance dripping blood, which was, of course, what the audience had paid to see. Ironically, fellow performers didn't realize it had happened, as they were all wearing blindfolds! We did consider trepanation – having holes bored in the skull on the road to enlightenment – but even the self-styled hardmen of British theatre wilted at the sight of a Dutch acid freak with a Black & Decker!

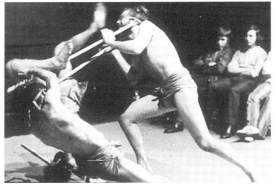

• *Blindfold*, RAT Theatre, 1973. Photo: Steve Allison

I want to tell you about *The Lesson of Anatomy*, a performance in four sections based on Artaud's various writings about the body – the body physical, the body social, the body spiritual, the body transcendental – presented by Cardiff Laboratory Theatre at Oval House in London early in 1974. I performed the first section, which was called *Flesh*. First time I ever shaved my head, as an artistic statement then of course, not the last hope of a balding, middle-aged man! Sitting on a marble slab, exposing bits of my anatomy as if for dissection – patient, specimen, case-study. Of the text, all I recall is 'All writing is pig-shit!', read from the label on my jacket pocket.

I want to … but I can barely remember. It's all so long ago and there's so little to help me. For this work – marginal, ephemeral, disposable – was never recorded, documented, analysed, held up for scrutiny. All that survives – the *traces* which devised performance leaves behind – is a few scars, the odd photograph, an occasional anecdote….

So instead, I want to tell you about my hero Peter Brötzmann.

I've always believed in writing to my heroes: letters to Eugenio Barba, John Berger, Test Dept, La Fura dels Baus, all resulted in creative collaboration.

Peter is a German saxophonist, one of the fathers of 'free music'. His 1968 album *Machine Gun* influenced a generation of European improvisers. In the 1980s, his music achieved a much wider constituency through his work with New York producer Bill Laswell in thrash-jazz outfit Last Exit, once described as 'all the music you've ever heard in your life, played at the same time'.

Performance Research 3(2), pp.35-41 © Routledge 1998

Peter's music thrills me, as no theatre can. For me, it all started with jazz, then jazz and poetry, then physical performance. As Walter Pater once wrote, 'All art constantly aspires towards the condition of music'.

Over the past few years Peter and I have worked regularly together as a duo. Our relationship started inauspiciously. We arranged to meet in Hamburg. Peter was late, too drunk to get on the train from Wuppertal. On the first afternoon, I decided to show him my 'principles of practice': how I could take a movement, invest it with more or less energy, make it tense, do a percentage of it, do it backwards. . . . At one point I caught him rolling his eyes heavenward! He had no need or desire to know my strategies. So, we just decided to go to work; two hours later we had made the opening part of our first performance *Der Gefesselte/The Bound Man*! You see, Peter has no concept of

rehearsing; when he's playing, he's playing. And he never plays less than 100 per cent. He once broke a rib blowing! Any rehearsal can be as good – whatever that means – as any performance. He always plays with fearsome energy and authority. He has no option. He is at the centre of his music, even if he is never at the middle of the note. He plays how he feels; his music is his voice. He is at heart a singer, 'a tooler of breath, his horn a long and strangely shaped larynx'. He generates immense breath but if he runs out, he just shouts or fingers the keys. As John Corbett has said:

> It would be difficult to imagine Brötzmann circular breathing, not only because it requires a technical conceit that goes against his anti-technical aesthetic, but because his basic unit is the breath. Every tone he makes he pushes forth with the motion of exhaling – giving sound the breath of life, bringing agitated life to each breath. And his phrasing is organised into breath-length lines; each of his statements is articulated with the capacity of his lungs, a finite, flesh-and-blood means of expression.*

* Sleeve notes to Brötzmann/Drake Duo *The Dried Rat-Dog* (Okka Disk OD12004 1995)

And in the great wave that hits you in heart and body, it's impossible to identify mistakes or bad bits.... As a collaborator, he's only interested in what you give, not the baggage, the history, the 'who-you've-trained-with', the 'who-you-know' that we carry as our identity card. I think he likes performing with me because although I'm obviously working, I don't crawl all over his music

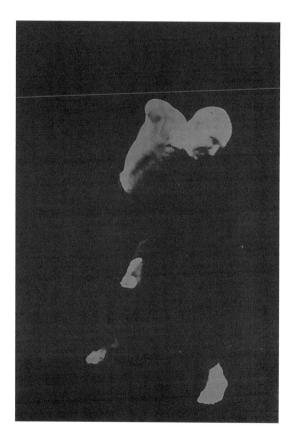

• *The Lesson of Anatomy*, Cardiff Laboratory Theatre, 1974. Photo: Steve Allison

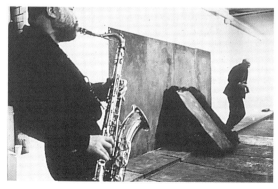

• *Der Gefesselte*, Brötzmann/Pearson, 1992. Photo: Andre Lützen

as every young-turk player, everyone who wants to blow him away, is wont to do!

What's it like? Well, you could buy the CD but you'd miss the physical engagement of the massive square head and great barrel chest. There is no score; no notation exists for this broken, slurred, dissonant music. It's no good asking Peter; he can't remember. He drinks before, during and after all rehearsals and performances. Your only option is to be there, in that protracted instant, that hour-long moment, where it exists, as nowhere else. Even memory fails, particularly with detail. Two hours later and all you remember is the physical experience. Any document is unintended. And as Peter rarely listens to his own recordings, it is also, for him, irrelevant.

Peter Brötzmann is 55 years old. He makes me feel so inadequate, so stupid. Our medium is so slow: training, conceptualizing, walk-throughs, technical rehearsal, dress rehearsal. Everything conspires to prevent us from doing it, our practice endlessly ensnared in strategical and tactical engagement, intention and operation, motives, stories, meanings…. I want to be more like Peter. I know we have contact, but oh, improv. But I begin to envisage something other. A conflation of impulse and action, energy and form, in the moment of execution.

I want to tell you about my friend Dave Levett.

Dave is a physical performer and computer musician: he controls his keyboard with his nose. When he was born, Dave was not breathing. This caused damage to his brain, affecting his motor functioning. Dave is neither mentally disabled, nor, as he is fed up of telling strangers who rush to his assistance in the street, is he deaf! Ten years ago he would have been called a spastic. Today he is regarded as 'having' – or 'suffering from' – cerebral palsy. In contemporary parlance he is 'disabled', not 'handicapped'.

Dave cannot stand unaided. Nevertheless, he generates tremendous pull and grip with his arms, and push with his legs. He refuses to use an electrically powered wheelchair, which he feels defines his 'status of dependency', and instead uses a standard manual chair, which he operates by pushing himself backwards with one foot. He cannot turn the wheels with his hands. Yet he achieves a precision of turn, spin, reverse, effectively with one toe. He communicates by laboriously pointing to a given vocabulary on a board on his lap or to individual letters to spell out more complex words. He also speaks, in gurgling tones. His voice, with its broken rhythms and swooping articulations – on the breath, against the breath – demands our attention, demands that we listen and interpret. And that we relax, that we accept that there is meaning here. His is a language that one has to learn. As his lungs don't inflate or deflate greatly, the nuances are subtle and there is extreme brevity and clarity in his words. Which is why he likes verbal puns so much.

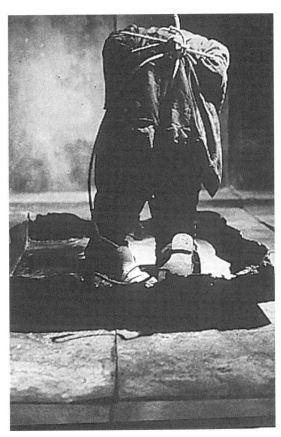

• *Der Gefesselte*, Brötzmann/Pearson, 1992. Photo: Andre Lützen

Five years ago we began to make physical theatre together. The rehearsal process meant the daily breaking of taboos. How do I touch a disabled man? How do I hold him? Will I damage him? Three moments I remember clearly from our early work :

– I was on my hands and knees. Dave was kneeling beside me. His action was to throw his body over mine. I remember his hand on my back and the enormous force of will as he imagined his goal and ordered his physical effort, and time, in a supreme effort of catching the moment. The feeling of organizing the body, directly experienced by those of us who hold and touch him in performance.

– I once dropped him. And he fell like a stone. Fortunately his body is tough. But he has no defence, no protective mechanism. To work with Dave is to know total responsibility.

– After the first performance, the audience was clearly moved. But not by Dave's disability. He despises pity and self-pity. By the fact that they realized that they knew what he meant. Yet he was not making anything close to a conventional gesture, rather a hovering net of gestural hint and suggestion. But with him isolated on the bare stage, with no redundancy of action on his part and no wavering of attention on our part, with a deep and extraordinary concentration, a will to communicate, to be understood, we experience him 'as signing', signalling through the flames perhaps. Exotic, fascinating, irresistible…. We are attracted by his humanity, by his heat …

Dave's body is in a kind of rebellion with itself, suddenly jerking into spastic movement or channelling creative impulse into stereotyped gesture. His body is *decided*. Yet he works with the actions his body wants to make. So 'pull' can become embrace, hold, grip, fight, tear. And 'push' becomes caress, reject, threaten. Or he can hitch a ride on the randomness and fury of physical abandon –

shaking, jerking, spasm-ing. He once told me that the one thing he can never do on stage is die, some part of his body is always in motion. His fingers always want to trace the most intricate and delicate of patterns. Yet just occasionally he can give a deep sigh and achieve the most awesome and terrible of silences. This is a dance of impulses: intended, random and spasmodic.

In our duet *In Black and White,* Dave worked both in and out of his chair. In *D.O.A.*, the chair was nowhere to be seen: Dave worked on a bed, on the floor, supported and carried by his two colleagues.

For me, Dave's work begins to pose fundamental questions about the nature of physical performance. What is the distinction between ability and disability, for his body can adopt positions, engage in actions which mine never can? What is the purpose and nature of training for the disabled

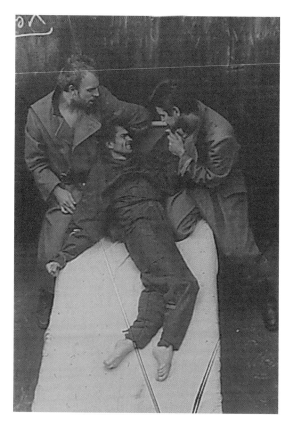

• *D.O.A.*, Brith Gof with Dave Levett, 1993. Photo: Mike Pearson

body which will never achieve athleticism? What does a notion such as choreography mean to the disabled performer? Or timing and dynamic, when action is the result of chance and will? Can the work of the disabled performer be confined by stylistic labels such as melodrama? Is 'what it is' as significant as 'what it portrays'?

Dave's work is impossible to notate; it resists the document. We will never come close to understanding his strategies. Only he will ever know what it feels like. We can never train to be like him. And video is not sophisticated enough to see the delicacy of hand gestures or the micro-movements of face and eye which communicate his precision of emotion and dramatic intent.

Both Peter and Dave work in, and with, the moment. They are the true heirs of Artaud: in relation to their work, all writing *is* pig shit. My association with them is causing me to reconsider the nature of my own work … and the status of documentation.

I begin to feel uneasy.

I feel uneasy that the demand for the document is part of a process of legitimization that is turning our practice into an orthodoxy and our life-wishes into a profession. As more and more university drama departments turn their attention to performance studies we begin to seek academic approbation and authentification. At best, this might cause us to be reasonable, rational, logical about work that is naturally none of these things. At worst, it may begin to represent a proprietorial struggle as to who is authorized to speak about, and for, the work and in what terms. And how ironic that more and more academic attention begins to focus upon less and less work.

For me, it's always been a political project. When I started with RAT Theatre in 1972, our work was a critique of the torpid youth culture – shrouded in a dope haze, 'flapping in flares' – of which we were part. We were fuelled by a set of attitudes to the body physical and the body politic; our gobs were full of situationist slogans. If we had been able to play guitars, we would have formed a band.

Instead, we made physical theatre – aggressive, violent, disturbing, ugly stuff – form and content locked in one semi-coherent outburst of energy. Theatre was our only option, but at least it was *ours*. No training, no teachers, no peers…. Arrogance, bad attitude, maximum exposure and effect. I feel uneasy turning performance into an object of study. I can teach technique but not attitude. We need more passion and less pedagogy. More dumb insolence in the face of those twin pillars of theatre – tradition and prudence – which refuse to tumble. The means will always follow the motive.

I feel uneasy.

I fear that theatre is already an anachronism: speedier media have already got 'replication' and 'representation' sown up. And performed behaviours, social simulations and staged events may already be happening in sophisticated ways elsewhere, not least in everyday life. In an era of surveillance, we are all constantly 'on stage'.

I feel uneasy.

I can no longer sit passively in the dark watching a hole in the wall, pretending that the auditorium is a neutral vessel of representation. It is a spatial machine that distances us from the spectacle and that allies subsidy, theatre orthodoxy and political conservatism, under the disguise of nobility of purpose, in a way that literally 'keeps us in our place'. I can no longer dutifully turn up to see the latest 'brilliant' product of such-and-such in this arts centre, where I saw the latest 'brilliant' product of others only yesterday, a field ploughed to exhaustion. I can no longer allow the programming policies and the black boxes of a circuit of venues to define the form and nature of performance.

I feel uneasy.

I have an urgent need to readdress my practice, to challenge and dismantle my own notions. Jerzy Grotowski's early work was dedicated to finding an authentic communication between one performer and one spectator – spatially, physically, emotionally. I imagine that he got up one morning and realized that the single thing which prevented such communication was theatre. And that's when he left. It will require that clarity of vision.

So what do I want ?

I want to get rid of the theatre 'object', the play, the 'well-made show', the *raison d'être* of the critic. I want to constitute performance as a strip of anti-social behaviour and incoherent activity, as a 'special world' where extra-daily occurrences and experiences and changes in status are possible.

I want to constitute performance as a 'field' of activity that will tend to escape definition, description and representation, there being no singular or external vantage point from which to view it. I want to create 'radically unfinished work', awkward, uneasy stuff which defies commodification as the latest product to buy, sell, hype in Europe.

I want to dislocate and confound the preconceptions, expectations and critical faculties of the audience. I want to problematize and renegotiate all three basic performance relationships: performer to performer, performer to spectator (and vice versa), and spectator to spectator. Standing, moving, running with, running away…. So that we may have to ask, 'Who is who?', 'Whom do I watch?', 'What's going on here?'

I want to find different arenas for performance – places of work, play and worship – where the laws and bye-laws, the decorum and learned contracts of theatre can be suspended.

I want to make performances that fold together place, performance and public.

I want to make 'hybrids' – of music, action, text and site – that defy conventional labels.

I want to make slippery, sliding performances that are not a mirror of some social issue or a simplification but a complication, which defies instant scrutiny.

And I want to reduce the critic to bystander.

I want to constitute performance as a discontinuous and interrupted practice of different modes of expression, of varying types and intensities, in which different orders of narrative can run simultaneously, in which dramatic concept may spring

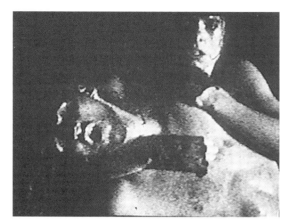

• *Gododdin*, Brith Gof, 1989.

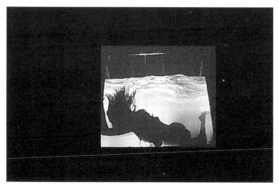

• *Pax*, Brith Gof, 1991.

from site, not story, and which may include rapid changes in mode and material.

What sort of traces will this leave? Where will the document reside?

If we are ridding ourselves of the 'critical object' then we can begin to characterize the event, the real-time manifestation, as a locus of experiences – spatial, physical and emotional. We can stop trying to reveal structure, the equivalent of dramatic script and emblem of authentification, and indeed what it means, what it's about. For my intentions will never be totally explicit. My practice is a kind of hidden knowledge articulated in a language which you will never understand. Just as I will never comprehend the baggage, more or less disguised, which you bring to my image. We must begin to deal with 'what it is', not 'what it might have been' or even 'what it resembles'.

Instead, we might concentrate on the sensual experiences of its individual agents, performance preserved in the bodies and memories of its varying orders of participants?. Touch, proximity, texture . . .

What are the extra-daily experiences, the suspensions of personal decorum?

What are the encounters and movements, the episodes and passings?

What are the implicit structures of inciting incidents and their trajectories, re-engagements, crises, irrevocable acts, sequences of tension, relaxation and acceleration, changes of consequence and innovation, ruptures and sudden shifts in direction and emphasis. What are the internal landmarks, the tactical engagements?

How is it characterized as 'easy bits', 'exciting sections', 'bloody hard work'?

How is it remembered as a pattern of body orientations, as a chain of demeanours, as a series of engagements of body to surface, to object, to environment?

How does it alter the perceptions and life strategies of its participants?

How is it preserved as analect and anecdote, description and incoherent babbling? A chorus of voices where the 'wagga, wagga, wagga' of the first-time heavy metal fan is no less authentic than the offended cries of the critic whose world is coming to pieces in *his* hands.

So that we find a 'way of telling' about it which has personal and communal currency. So that we can endlessly replay it, thrill again to it, enshrine it in our mythology …

So that perhaps, in the end, the best we can ever do is to ask, 'How was it for you?' Which probably tells you quite a lot about Antonin Artaud and me.

Versions of this provocation were presented at the Centre for Performance Research/Lancaster University Summer School of Theatre symposium 'Mind The Gaps'/Performance: Process and Documentation, Lancaster, England, July 1994 and at the Centre for Performance Research symposium 'Past Masters: Antonin Artaud', Aberystwyth, Wales, November 1996.

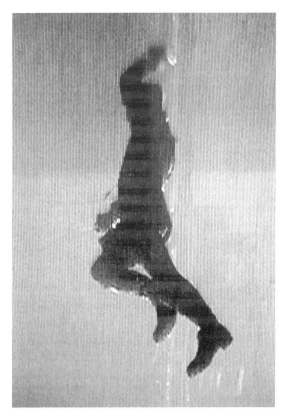

• *Haearn*, Brith Gof, 1992.

Re-Languaging the Body: Phenomenological Description and the Dance Image

Nigel Stewart

1 'I' AM 'IT'

Consciousness

I want to write about writing about moving. How can I re-language the body and re-embody writing so that I can reawaken the sensations of dancing and not merely register the social implications of dance? How can language probe the relation between the subjective life of the dancer and the objective form of the dance? Phenomenology furthers this inquiry because it reflects upon the dialectic between subject and object, the 'I' who perceives and the 'It' or 'Thou' which is apperceived. On the one hand, phenomenology presupposes that consciousness is always *intentional,* which is to say that 'consciousness . . . has an object – that consciousness is a *consciousness of something*' (Fraleigh 1987: 6). However, phenomenology equally presupposes that objects 'can only be apprehended subjectively' (*OED*, sense b). It claims that the object of which we are conscious is the object *as it appears to us* through our faculty of intuition (or sympathy). Phenomenology suggests methods for intuiting *phenomena* (or objects as we perceive them) within the sensible sphere of our lived experience.

However, if phenomenology avoids the objectivist fallacy it equally refuses to collapse into mere subjectivism, that is, the 'radically personal and situational theory of value' based on the belief 'that I can make anything out of the objects I perceive', a view growing from 'atheistic existentialism' and 'culminati[ng] in pathological narcissism' (Fraleigh 1987: 96, 139). In fact, phenomenology recognizes that objects have an *inherent* value (i.e. a capacity to elicit an aesthetic response), even if it insists that 'the process of valuing is founded experientially in subjectivity' (ibid.: 45). For instance, phenomenological aesthetics argues that subjective feeling does not exist prior to the object of the art work. Feeling does not seek a form to express itself through. On the contrary, feeling is *produced in and through* the contemplation or performance of the art work. Feeling is the *gestalt intimated* (not *imitated*) by a work's aesthetic form (Goodman 1968: 46–53).

Yet aesthetic form will fully exist only when *it has been experienced subjectively as it is realized physically*. The choreographic form of the dance work, for instance, is alive only when it has been 'dissolved (realized) in action' by the dancer (Fraleigh 1987: 21). But if the dance will be a dance only when it is danced, this happens only when (usually through assiduous training and rehearsal) the dance has been learnt so well that it becomes the dancer's second nature. Even the will and effort

Performance Research 3(2), pp.42–53 © Routledge 1998

to create or perform the work has to 'sink back into nature' (ibid.: 20). If I instruct my arm to rise my arm is *not* dancing. It is only when I feel the practised neuromuscular pathway through which my arm is already rising that I have a dancing arm. Paradoxically, volitional action feels spontaneous because it has sunk deep into my body. In such moments 'voluntary motion of the body does not present itself as a native power of an *imperium* over an inert body, but as a dialogue with a bodily spontaneity' (Ricoeur 1966: 227). When this occurs the dance object *is* the moving conscious subject. The dancer is the dance. 'I' am 'It':

> The body is not something I possess to dance with. I do not order my body to bend here and whirl there. I do not think 'move,' then do move. No! I am the dance; its thinking is its doing and its doing is its thinking. I am the bending and I am the whirling. My dance is my body as my body is myself.
>
> (Fraleigh 1987: 32)

Kinaesthesia

In fact, with the existential phenomenology of Sartre (1956) and Merleau-Ponty (1962[1945]), phenomenology has insisted that intentional consciousness is *always already* a bodily event (Bachelard 1964[1958]: xv; States 1992: 370, 375–6). Vital support for this view is offered by the sensory psychology of Gibson (1968). In effect, Gibson challenged the old idea of sensation as merely the internal effect of an external cause. The image theory of the ancient Greeks proposed that an object emitted a faint image of itself and that the senses were merely passive channels through which the image of an object was transmitted to the mind or *sensorium*. '[T]hey believed', therefore, 'that sensations derived *directly* from the properties of external objects' (Reason 1982: 219). This belief was critiqued by philosophers and scientists from the seventeenth century onwards but persisted until Johannes Müller formulated his famous doctrine of specific nerve energies in 1826. Müller's basic assertion (consistent with phenomenology's epistemology of the object) was that we can never

directly experience the qualities of an object, only the *qualities (or energies) of the sensory nerves* as they are excited by that object. According to Müller, each nerve has a specific energy corresponding to one of the classical five senses (Reason 1982: 220).

Müller's doctrine was the basis of Sherrington's widely used classification of the senses (1973[1906]). In Sherrington's system a surface sheet of *exteroceptors* (receptors joining the external world, such as the eyes, ears, nose, mouth and skin) and *interoceptors* (receptors in the alimentary canal and visceral organs) cover a deep cellular field of *proprioceptors* (receptors in the inner ear, muscles, tendons and joints). Sherrington thus argued for a sixth, proprioceptive or *kinaesthetic* sense – the sensation producing awareness of movement and the position of body parts. None the less, Sherrington's system, like Müller's doctrine, did not counter the fundamental assumption that sensation is always 'the *result* of the action of an *external cause*' (Müller 1948[1838]: 162; emphasis added).

By contrast, Gibson showed that the six senses are more active in their engagement with the external world and more interactive in their engagement with each other. Gibson's alternative classificatory system cross-referred two types of sensation (*exteroception* or the detection of environmental events, and *proprioception* or the detection of bodily events) with two types of stimulation (the *imposed* where the senses provide *passive channels of sensation*, and the *obtained* where proprioception and exteroception *actively gather information*). '[W]e are', then, 'not merely passive observers subject to the imprint of the surrounding world. Consciousness selects, sorts out, and organizes stimuli according to present purposeful perception – purposeful because it is directed toward, and involved in, its objects. The body, in this view, is a sensitive perceptive actor. It does not *have* a consciousness – rather it *is* a consciousness' (Fraleigh 1987: 15).

But Gibson went further. The problem with Sherrington's classification, he argued, was 'the fallacy of ascribing proprioception to propriocep-tors' (Gibson 1968: 33). In fact '[w]e obtain a sense of our own movement not only from specialized [proprioceptive] receptors in the inner ear, joints, tendons and muscles, but also from what we can see, hear and feel. . . . Vision', for instance, 'is kinaesthetic in that it registers movements of the body just as much as do the vestibular receptors and those in the muscles, joints and skin' (Reason 1982: 223). Contrary to Sherrington's direct corre-lation of sensory experience with the activation of specific receptors and their nerves at different cellular levels, the kinaesthetic sense is a gestalt emerging from the *interaction* of all the *other* senses. After Gibson we can speak of kinaesthesia in terms of its muscular, articular, vestibular, cutaneous, auditory and visual modalities (Gibson 1968: 36–8). In this view, kinaesthesia is the ground to our con-sciousness.

Creating Time and Space

All this is fuel to the phenomenologist's fire. The Gibsonian classification of sensation and stimu-lation not only supports phenomenology's notion of consciousness as, by definition, an intentional *corporeal* consciousness, but also supports dance phenomenology's concern with describing con-sciousness in terms of the structure of the sensation of the *moving* body. Such a body opposes mere '*flesh*, the body not infused with life but dragged around' (Sparshott 1984: 188). On the contrary, the body which *is* our active intentional consciousness consists of the 'congeries of sense' of what Merleau-Ponty called 'the lived body' (Cohen 1984: 164) – the body as a 'moving form . . . not distin-guished from the consciousness and character of the embodied person' (Sparshott 1984: 188).

This has three vital implications for our under-standing of the dance image. First, we cannot

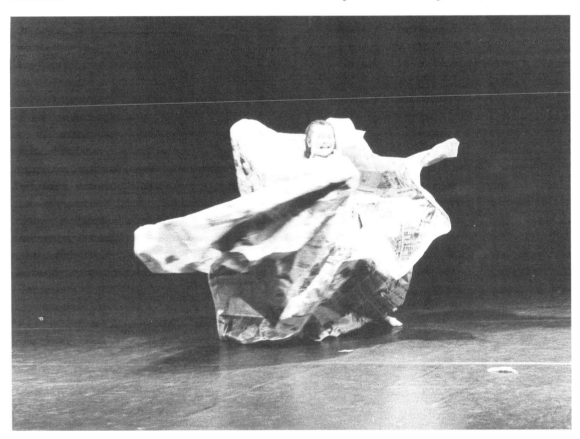

Natsu Nakajima, 10th ISTA, Copenhagen, 1996. Photo: Fiora Bemporad

pronounce on the space and time of the dance as if they are objects that can be set apart from the sensations of the space and time of the subject who dances. We can, however, speak of the space of the dance as it is created and moulded by the dancer (Deborah Jowitt, cit. in Fraleigh 1987: 181). The dancer, then, does not merely *inhabit* space: 'to be a body, is to be tied to a certain world, our body is not primarily *in* space: it is *of* it' (Merleau-Ponty, cit. in Fraleigh 1987: 178).

Second, if dance phenomenology is primordially concerned with the form of the body-in-motion then this is, *ipso facto*, a form-in-time, a *form-in-the-making*. We cannot then consider the dancer's body as if it is stuck in a static temporality, an externally related series of discrete moments (like photographic images) or of psychic states and actions. On the contrary, we will want to consider the dance image in terms of the *dynamic temporality of the moving body*. According to Gibson we can proactively derive kinaesthetic information from static visual objects (such as the photograph), but until that information is itself integrated as the felt trajectory of a moving force we will not grasp the dance image. '[P]hotographs', then, 'are not dance images – they are photographic images of the dance' (Fraleigh 1987: 210). Rather, the dance image is *diasporatic* – 'a temporal structure whose meaning derives only from the interrelationship of its units' (Sheets-Johnstone 1979: 18). The body grows and flows through time. The body bleeds beyond the static sign. It smudges and stands out from any frozen representation of itself. This is the 'body-in-life' (Barba 1988), the body in 'flight'. This is the falling body, the body in *'ecstasis* [within which] *temporality temporalizes itself as . . . the structural whole of existence*' (Heidegger 1962: 401–3; cf. Sheets-Johnstone 1979: 16).

Third, if we are dealing with consciousness as it is *presencing* itself as the moving body, we are dealing only with that very *instant* at which we perceive the object as an image of which we are conscious. Now a cultural materialist would claim that this phenomenal image is 'always tainted by a lifetime of perceptual habit within a narrow

cultural frame'. A semiotician would claim that the *image* (as something which is nothing but itself), is inevitably turned by socialized codification into a *sign* (something which substitutes for something else), or that the meaning of that sign 'retreat[s] . . . before the finger of definition' (as something always becoming something else). A phenomenologist, however, reflects upon the pre-reflective sensation of the image – 'the Big Bang' of 'the perceptual explosion' (States 1992: 370, 374).

Phenomenological description thus involves *eidetic* analysis (i.e., stemming from the detailed and exceptionally vivid recall of sensuous imagery) as a mode of epistemological inquiry which seeks to reconstruct philosophy 'on the pared-down but firm foundations of a knowledge in and of the world' (Norris 1982: 44). For this reason, the systematically analytical phenomenology of Husserl, the founder of phenomenology, depends on the *epoché*, the subject's capacity to 'bracket' or 'reduce' an object by discounting the object's actual existence and the accident of impressions that surrounds it. The subject can then apprehend the basic and *constitutive structures through which the object is perceived*. Phenomenological reduction thus demands that we strip the object of 'layer upon layer of culturally derived preconceptions and predispositions [that] obscure a direct view of life and of the life-world' (Fallico 1962: 7). Phenomenology is therefore not just the 'science of appearances' (Vesey and Foulkes 1990: 220); it is the science of essences deduced from appearances. Accordingly, dance phenomenology reduces the dance image to *the structures intrinsic and essential to our sensations of the moving body*. The dance image is therefore finally a 'significant form' *without a socialized significance*:

> The basic concept is the *articulate but non-discursive form having import without conventional reference*, and therefore presenting itself *not as a symbol in the ordinary sense, but as a 'significant form,'* in which the factor of significance is not logically discriminated, but is felt as a *quality* rather than recognized as a [semantic] *function*.
>
> (Langer 1953: 32; emphasis added)

2 DESCRIPTIONS

'Forcetimespace'

Dance phenomenology elucidates the spatial and temporal structures intrinsic to the subject's lived experience of the *force* (energy or *bios*) which is revealed in a specific dance. We can systematically reflect upon a *temporalization of force* (the tensional and projectional qualities of the dance) and a *spatialization of force* (linear and areal qualities).*

Moreover, we can deepen this reflection by detailing the dynamics of the moving body using Laban Motif Writing, particularly as it has been developed in the Language of Dance from structured Labanotation (Hutchinson Guest 1985; Hutchinson Guest 1996). We can consider dynamics in terms of, say, the body's *flow* in space, that is, 'the degree of liberation produced in movement' (Laban 1980[1950]: 75) considered in relation to central and peripheral space (Hutchinson Guest 1985: 7).†

It is, however, only in the specific interplay of spatial and temporal qualities that force is revealed:

> What we see is something which perhaps can only be empirically written as forcetimespace; an indivisible wholeness appears before us. Space, time, and force are certainly apparent in dance, but they are not and cannot be objectively apparent. To conceive of them as given objective factors beforehand is to overlook the very quiddity of dance: it is

* *Tensional qualities* are determined by the amount of effort that the body is perceived to be exerting. *Projectional qualities* are decided by the manner in which force is projected (abrupt, sustained, etc.). *Linear qualities* trace the cumulative process or growth of motion (Langer 1953: 65–6). Linear qualities have a design and a pattern: the *linear design* is the shape of the imaginary line which runs through the body (e.g. curved, twisted, etc.); the *linear pattern* is the imaginary line which the body traces as it travels through space (straight, circular, etc.), usually in relation to a focal point. Areal qualities also have a design and a pattern: the *areal design* is the perceptual form and perceived size or amplitude of the body as a centre of force (contractive, expansive, etc.); the *areal pattern* is the perceptual form and amplitude of the (stage) space that surrounds the body and the imaginary texture of that space (resistant, pliant, etc.) through which force is projected (Sheets-Johnstone 1979: cc. 4, 9).

† Motif Writing therefore aids phenomenological inquiry in so far as it perceives and documents not just quantitative data, but such 'subtle [qualitative] distinctions; in this way, the notation can be consistent with the particular conceptualization of the movement' (Youngerman 1984: 114).

something which is created and which does not exist prior to its creation.

> (Sheets-Johnstone 1979: 14; cf. Sheets-Johnstone 1984: 135)

The Expressive Figure

But there is more to be said. As I systematically describe the structures intrinsic to my lived experience (as dancer or spectator) of the dance, I slide into a kind of revelry which is far from systematic. I begin to daydream the dance. Within this daydream my kinaesthetic sensation of dancing condenses and deepens. Now this sensation gives rise to what I will generally call an *expressive figure*. The figure can take various forms. It can be a poetic word or series of words or an abstract graphic mark – but it is always birthed by and absolutely intrinsic and specific to the 'forcetimespace' of my dancing body or the dancer's body which I apperceive.

In fact I want to suggest that a phenomenological description of the 'forcetimespace' of the dance image reaches fruition only when systematic reflection generates expressive (poetic or figural) forms of writing and the systematic and the expressive are combined in consciousness.

At this crucial juncture I want to investigate three praxes (or models of practice) of expressive writing. Each praxis provides a different example of one of the expressive figures to which I have alluded – but all three enlarge our understanding and experience of the image of the moving body and therefore count as phenomenological descriptions of dance. They are ways of writing *about* the dancing body *from* the dancing body.

Hijikata's Notation System

Phenomenology is happier with the 'essentially *variational*' nature of the poetic image than with the '*constitutive*' nature of the concept (Bachelard 1964[1958]: xv), and the poetic image is precisely the kind of expressive figure central to the 'double notation system' of Tatsumi Hijikata who founded Butoh with Kazuo Ohno over thirty years ago. Hijikata's notation system is a praxis in which, in effect, bodily energy can be imaged and modulated through a poetic subtext.

It works like this: each action is given a poetic title and placed with at least one other action in a unit or phrase of actions. These larger phrases are in turn given titles and arranged into the whole composition. The title for each action evokes a bodily sensation intrinsic to the action rather than a concept which can be extrapolated from it. Similarly, the title for each phrase suggests not a theme which runs through the actions but the elemental energy quality – or what Hijikata called the 'space power' – which governs them. An example is provided by the dance *Sleep of Stone* (Hijikata 1996), which I witnessed in a performance by Natsu Nakajima, Hijikata's disciple. In *Sleep of Stone* there are nine phrases (Sleep; Flower; Willow and Wind; Sleep of Stone; Willow; Orchard; Willow and Smoke; Stuffed Air; and The Action of Hands), each containing a succession of up to seventeen actions. In Stuffed Air there are two actions. In the first action, 'Hands and Nail', Nakajima's trunk tilts towards forward-high and twists to the right from the waist.* The right arm simultaneously extends to left-side-middle in front of the left arm which remains flexed as it inclines towards left-forward-low. She faces forward-middle, baring her teeth. 'Hands and Nail' then slowly mutates into the subsequent configuration, 'A Hawk', in which the whole of the trunk extends further to parallel the floor, whilst the arms spread laterally, each to its own side-middle.

It would be possible to read the acts of a predator into Nakajima's performance, but, especially given the absence of a narrative context, the emphasis is far more on the abstract energetic quality of her actions and less on what they might signify. Using the systematic criteria of dance phenomenology and Language of Dance I can observe that 'Hands and Nail' emphasizes more the motion and less the destination of the action, whilst 'A Hawk' is the opposite. However, the two configurations have shared qualities. They both have a sustained projection, firm tension, resistant spatial texture and bound energy flow, and muscular control with a central inner attitude. These qualities common to

* This method of reference is based on Laban's kinesphere. It is incorporated in Laban Motif Writing which I used to make notes during Nakajima's performance. For a comprehensive account of direction and other concepts and the symbols through which they are notated in Laban Motif Writing see Hutchinson Guest 1995 and Laban 1966: 13–17.

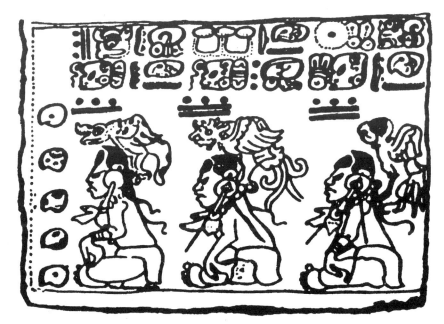

Fig. 1 A Mayan graphic complex, combining hieroglyphic text (top), number signs (a dot = 1, a hyphen = 5) and a pictogram (bottom). Credit: V. Istrine, *Origine et développement de l'écriture*

the two actions define the particular 'space power' governing the phrase. *But I only fully intuit the 'forcetimespace' of this dance image when I allow my systematic reflections on the qualities of the phrase to sink into a kinaesthetic meditation on the expressive figure Stuffed Air.*

Ancient Graphic Writing

Hijikata's poetic titles compare, in my view, with the various figures used in ancient graphic writing in that both trace physical sensation. In Sumerian, for instance, the logogram for 'water' was two horizontal parallel undulating lines. In Chinese, 'pipe' is written not by representing the object but by tracing the gesture that designates it, whilst the Chinese hieroglyph for 'friend' is the design of two interlocking hands (Kristeva 1989 [1981]: 24–5).

In other graphic systems the movement of the microcosmos is traced in relation to the macrocosmos. In Mayan, for example, pictograms (outlining people, heads, arms, gestures, animals, plants, artefacts, and so on) were composed with hieroglyphic text and number signs into 'graphic complexes' lined by a square or circle, thus suggesting 'the inclusion and pulverization of the signifying "subject" in a divided and ordered cosmos' (ibid.: 61; cf. Fig. 1). In a similar way the maps of Renaissance Ptolemaic cosmogony related bodily organs and humours to the elements and signs of the zodiac (Evans 1987: ill. 28–30). Therefore, 'for primitive man [*sic*] . . . language is not . . . an abstract thought process. It . . . is joined with the motor force of the body and nature' (Kristeva 1989 [1981]: 50).

The Hieroglyphs of Contact Improvisation

Nancy Stark Smith, a co-founder of Contact Improvisation, has likewise experimented with hieroglyphic figures that express the body's motor force (cf. Fig. 2). In fact, Laban observed that the trace forms (or linear patterns) of bodily movement always consist of combinations of straight, curved, twisted and rounded lines and that 'the best way to

convince oneself of this fact is to scribble on a piece of paper, in one uninterrupted line' (Laban 1966: 83). Moreover, trace forms can be considered not just as a kind of writing but as *dynamospheric* writing if we understand the dynamosphere in terms of the dynamic created from peripheral trace forms working with and against the 'hidden content' of central 'shadow forms' (e.g. subtle inclinations of the head, hands, or torso) (ibid.: 90–1). Comparably, improvisation exercises in postmodern dance classes frequently envisage dancing as mark-making:

EXERCISE Imagine a writing instrument is located at the top of your head, at the soft spot where the bones of the skull meet. Imagine you can draw with this instrument as a sky-writing plane draws in space. The space around you is a three-dimensional canvas. Allow your writing instruments to draw pathways on the canvas, letting the rest of your body be loose and responsive. Adjust your body to accommodate your drawing pathways, always letting the

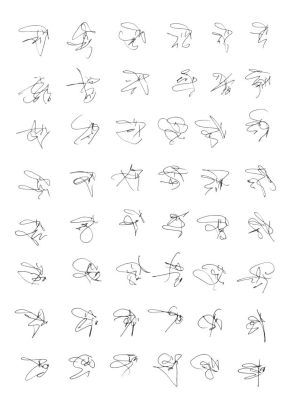

Fig. 2 Nancy Stark Smith, Hieroglyphs, 1988.

48

top of your head lead. Explore different speeds, levels, and degrees of locomotion. Allow your eyes to scan, seeing all but focusing on nothing. Work to the point of disorientation and stop.

(Gamble 1977: 38)

The linear patterns seen and felt in such exercises flow into the 'writing thriving lines' of Smith's hieroglyphic marks. 'Suspended, as if in mid air directly above the page, the hieroglyphs dwell in a nebulous space somewhere between dancing and writing, where the movements of the one influence the rhythm and figures of the other.' The lines, curved lines, double waves and rounded lines, swishes, swirls, swerves and loops of Smith's hieroglyphs encircle and create spaces – but more importantly there is a vital crack in the line that allows the inner space to leak out into the wider space, generating an *ekstasis* across the page beyond the marks themselves (Albright 1989: 49a).

Re-Languaging the Body

I will now make this claim: Hijikata's titles, ancient graphics and Smith's hieroglyphs not only count as forms of phenomenological description, but lead to some otherwise unattainable conclusions about the phenomenal dance image.

First, these three forms of expressive writing aid phenomenological inquiry in that they probe in various ways the complex relationship between the object of the dance and the subject who dances. Certainly, these ways of notating movement directly flow from the sensations of moving. Smith, for example, observes that her hieroglyphs 'precisely capture the frequency of [her] mood, mind and body rhythm', and that the 'connections' she 'found . . . between . . . dancing and the movement of [her] pen' were so 'direct' that she sees both as forms of 'signature' (Smith 1982: 45c, 46b).

These expressive forms also reflect the *way* in which the imaginary or actual objects through which movement is notated (e.g. stuffed air, flowing water, interlocking hands, canvas lines) flow from

and into the subject's movement. They *mark* the very manner in which the object is kinaesthetically perceived by, and danced from, the subject's consciousness. So, from one point of view, these forms of notation embody a unity – prized by phenomenology – between the *dancing* subject and the object that is *danced* and reciprocally compels the subject to *dance*:

[T]he dancer [does not] adopt movement[s] or attitudes to *simulate* something – for example a flower . . . the dancer actually transforms him/herself into a flower . . . *the dancer needs to believe* 'I'm a flower', or 'I'm a stone' more like [a child playing] or a medium in trance.

(Nakajima 1996: 2; emphasis added)

Moreover, the expressive figures used in these experimental or ancient writings implicitly liken the experiences of watching, notating and dancing a dance. All three expressive figures evoke a sensation of motion skidding beyond the figure. We have already noticed how Smith's hieroglyphs in particular generate an *ekstasis* beyond the hieroglyphs. Comparably, Hijikata's poetic images, and metaphors in general, '[operate] through words composed into full gestalts (phrases or images) that refer us to something beyond the words' (Fraleigh 1987: 171). However, this *ekstasis* occurs only if 'I' (the 'reader') allow myself to be kinaesthetically affected by 'It' (the expressive figure). These expressive figures then elicit in me an aesthetic response, which *re-enacts* the aesthetic response to movement of Hijikata, the ancient cultures, or Smith. To complete the circle, those notational responses are re-enactments of the dancer's aesthetic response to the object with which the movement is 'notated' and to which I respond. But whether I am reader, spectator, notator, or dancer, 'I' (the subject) have to embody 'It' (the object) by becoming kinaesthetically conscious of the image of the object. To this extent the object sinks into my nature. When this happens my being is my doing. If my doing is the aesthetic form of the dance (or the expressive writing through which the dance is notated) then my being is *enlarged* by and into the dance: 'to embody a dance involves a forming of our own *given* embodiment *toward* an *aesthetic* embodiment' (ibid.: 117; emphasis added). These expressive figures therefore betoken the self's 'new embodied meaning' with which phenomenological aesthetics is concerned (Reid 1969: 61).

When dance thus unites movement with being it brings the Closed of the Earth (that which has been 'unnoticed, or untapped' by the body) into the Open of the World (the aesthetic form). The form-in-the-making reveals the concealed (Fraleigh 1987: 89; Heidegger 1975). As we have especially seen with the Sumerian logogram for 'water' and the Chinese hieroglyphs for 'pipe' and 'friend', the expressive figure in general also unites our being with language by revealing the concealed *gestural* basis to language. It shows that movement 'subtends the word' (Fraleigh 1987: 86). Commensurately, it shows that 'language and body elements . . . start from the same big tree root' from which physical actions grow as the 'leaves of words' (Nakajima 1996: 6).

But if the expressive figures of Hijikata, Smith and the ancient or 'primitive' cultures advise that subject and object are always inextricably linked they equally suggest that subject and object are *distinguishable*. Indeed, Smith's experiments with hieroglyphs stem from her interest in 'what happens *between* [a pre-reflective] experience and the [reflective] telling of it' (Smith 1982: 45). She 'has sought not so much to bridge the gap between writing and dancing as to probe the space itself' (Albright 1989: 39a). If the subject is pre-reflectively involved in the object of the dance there is no gap between subject and object. However, when the subject reflects on a dance such a gap opens up. Recognition brings rupture. Now these expressive figures are tantalizingly and equivocally situated between the pre-reflective and the reflective. In so far as the expressive figure stems from kinaesthetic sensation and thus reawakens the subject's felt unity with the dance object, it feels, in part, the *same* as dancing. But these expressive figures are, of course, not *identical* with the dance. They are symbols of the felt life of the dance. Yet even as I

am aware of this *difference* between the expressive figure and the dance, I *experience the element of the same* in *the difference*. The figures of Hijikata, ancient graphics and Nancy Stark Smith thus '[work] with a logic of sameness *and* difference that quite outleaps the ordinary logic of contradiction, the ordinary logic of identity *or* exclusion' (Harland 1987: 139), to enter the realm of *différance*: 'the *same*, which is not the identical . . . [in] the diverted and equivocal passage from one difference to another, one term of the opposition to the other' (Derrida 1973: 148). Thus if I bemoan a *difference* between my reflection upon the dance and my pre-reflective sensation of dancing, the expressive figure can transmute that difference into a *différance* which inserts an element of the same (a similarity of sensation) into the element of difference (a position of distance). This 'disparity action' (Richards 1965), or rub between sameness and difference, produces an energy that evokes the very energy of dancing the dance. In this sense, the expressive figure operates in relation to the dance very much as one dancer does to another when dancing in unison: the experience of the *same* choreographic material in *different* bodies produces an energy greater than would be the case in a solo performance.

Finally, Hijikata's double notation system, ancient graphic writing and Smith's hieroglyphs have the same end as phenomenological reduction in that they intensify the felt life of movement and consequently delay the moment when the movement image is interpreted as a codified sign. We can theorize this in at least two ways. First, ancient graphics and Smith's hieroglyphs in particular compare with Kristeva's notion of the semiotic. Each consists of a 'distinct mark, trace, index . . . engraven or written sign, imprint' (Kristeva 1986: 93) with a 'kinetic rhythm' or 'pulsion' which 'pulls meaning away from its traditional moorings' (Albright 1989: 48b–49a).

Second, these ancient or experimental expressive figures coincide with the art symbol in general in that they are significant forms without socialized significance. They primarily have value in terms of

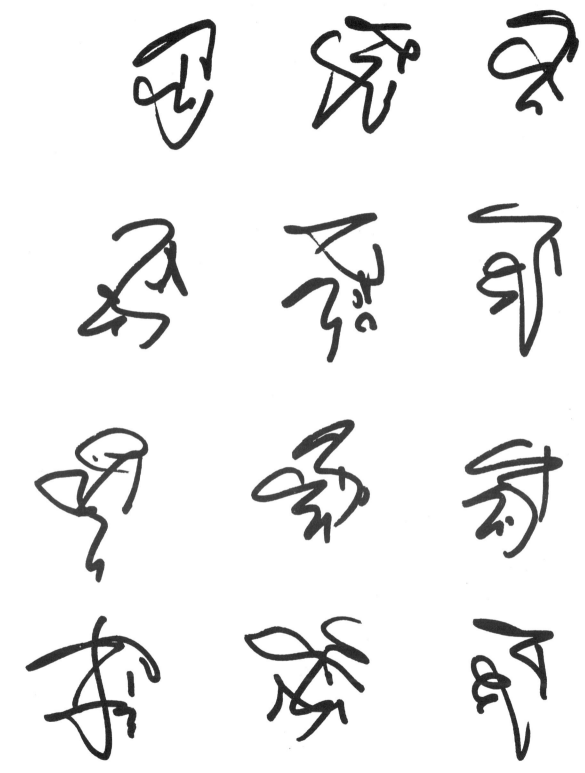

Fig. 3 Nancy Stark Smith, Hieroglyphs, 1998.

the physical sensations which they produce. They have no or little function outside of that context. In structuralist sign theory, these expressive figures would be best understood as *nonce symbols*, 'private one-off symbols, such as appear in dreams or in poetry, which convey no public information until they are provided with an additional gloss', unlike *standardized symbols* in which the form of the signifier is linked to the content of the signified by a wholly arbitrary but none the less conventional code fully understood 'in the public domain' (Leach 1976: 15). Thus 'it is very important for dancers to understand [Hijikata's] notation through their own physical sensations, not as a signal or code.' (Nakajima 1996: 5). Hijikata's titles, ancient graphics and Smith's hieroglyphs have, then,

> symbolic agency . . . so close to overt expression that it fairly shimmers. . . . But [their] real office here has nothing to do with the iconographic functions usually assigned to symbols in art. The artistic symbol, qua artistic, negotiates insight, not reference . . . It is deeper than any semantic of accepted signs and their referents, more essential than any schema that may be heuristically read.
>
> (Langer 1953: 22)

So in these three forms of expressive writing, poetic words or graphic marks must be understood as the dance image is understood in dance phenomenology: not as part of a process of systematic signification and mentalization abstracted from the body, but precisely as the possibility of delaying that process in order for the subject to re-experience the qualities and sensations of the body's energies in relation to the world and to modulate those energies in performance.

These praxes are phenomenological praxes in that they provide not verbal equivalents for energetic qualities but a process of 're-languaging' in which 'one must come to grips

* I would like to express my deep gratitude to Amanda Williamson, Professor Baz Kershaw and Dr Isis Brook for their meticulous responses to successive drafts of this article, and to Professor Maria Shevtsova and Richard Gough for providing helpful remarks on an earlier and much longer version. I would also like to pay tribute to Maxine Sheets-Johnstone and Sondra Horton Fraleigh for the paths they have cleared in the field of dance phenomenology and aesthetics.

linguistically with the phenomenon as it gives itself in experience' (Sheets-Johnstone 1984: 132, 135). Re-languaging invites a meditation on the experience of dancing that neither sacrifices the integrity and immediacy of that experience nor vitiates its intrinsic qualities (Sheets-Johnstone 1979: xii, xv). It keeps the live experience alive. It is the body's way of wor(l)ding the world.*

REFERENCES

Albright, Ann Cooper (1989) 'Writing the moving body: Nancy Stark Smith and the hieroglyphics', *Frontiers: A Journal of Women's Studies* X(3): 36–51.

Bachelard, Gaston (1964[1958]) *The Poetics of Space*, trans. Maria Jolas, foreword Etienne Gilson, Boston, MA: Beacon.

Barba, Eugenio (1988) 'The way of refusal: the theatre's body-in-life', *New Theatre Quarterly* IV(16): 291–9.

Cohen, Sibyl S. (1984) 'Ingarden's aesthetics and dance', in Maxine Sheets-Johnstone (ed.) *Illuminating Dance: Philosophical Explorations*, London: Associated University Presses, pp. 146–66.

Derrida, Jacques (1973) *Speech and Phenomena, and Other Essays on Husserl's Theory of Signs*, trans. David B. Allison, Evanston, IL: Northwestern University Press.

Evans, G. Blakemore (ed.) (1987) *Elizabethan-Jacobean Drama*, London: A. & C. Black.

Fallico, Arturo B. (1962) *Art and Existentialism*, Englewood Cliffs, NJ: Prentice-Hall.

Fraleigh, Sondra Horton (1987) *Dance and the Lived Body: A Descriptive Aesthetics*, Pittsburgh, PA: University of Pittsburgh Press.

Gamble, John (1977) 'On contact improvisation', *The Painted Bride Quarterly* IV(1).

Gibson, James J. (1968) *The Senses Considered as Perceptual Systems*, London: Allen & Unwin.

Goodman, Nelson (1968) *Languages of Art: An Approach to a Theory of Symbols*, Indianapolis, IN: Bobbs-Merrill.

Harland, Richard (1987) *Superstructuralism: The Philosophy of Structuralism and Post-Structuralism*, London: Methuen.

Heidegger, Martin (1962) *Being and Time*, trans. John Macquarrie and Edward Robinson, Oxford: Blackwell.

Heidegger, Martin (1975) 'The origin of the work of art', *Poetry, Language, Thought*, trans. Albert Hofstadter, New York: Harper & Row, pp. 15–87.

Hijikata, Tatsumi (chor.) (1996) *Sleep of Stone*, perf. Natsu Nakajima, 10th International School of Theatre Anthropology, Kanonhallen in Copenhagan, 4 May.

Hutchinson Guest, Ann (1985) 'Dynamics', *The Labanotator* 40.

Hutchinson Guest, Ann (1995) *Your Move: A New Approach to the Study of Movement and Dance*, New York and London: Gordon & Breach.

Hutchinson Guest, Ann (1996) 'What exactly do we mean by dynamics: Part One', *Dance Theatre Journal* XIII(2): 28–33.

Kristeva, Julia (1986) 'Revolution in poetic language', in Toril Moi (ed.) *The Kristeva Reader*, New York: Columbia University Press, pp. 90–136.

Kristeva, Julia (1989 [1981]) *Language the Unknown: An Initiation into Linguistics*, trans. Anne M. Menke, Hemel Hempstead, Herts: Harvester Wheatsheaf.

Laban, Rudolf (1966) *Choreutics*, ann. and ed. Lisa Ullmann, London: MacDonald & Evans.

Laban, Rudolf (1980 [1950]) *The Mastery of Movement*, rev. and enl. Lisa Ullmann, London: MacDonald & Evans.

Langer, Susanne K. (1953) *Feeling and Form: A Theory of Art Developed from Philosophy in a New Key*, London and Henley: Routledge & Kegan Paul.

Leach, Edmund (1976) *Culture and Communication: the Logic by which Symbols are Connected. An Introduction to the Use of Structuralist Analysis in Social Anthropology*, Cambridge: Cambridge University Press.

Merleau-Ponty, Maurice (1962 [1945]) *Phenomenology of Perception*, London: Routledge & Kegan Paul.

Müller, Johannes (1948 [1838]) 'The Specific Energies of Nerves', in Wayne Dennis (ed.) *Readings in the History of Psychology*, New York: Appleton-Century-Crofts, pp. 157–68.

Nakajima, Natsu (1996) untitled lecture paper, Copenhagen: International School of Theatre Anthropology.

Norris, Christopher (1982) *Deconstruction: Theory and Practice*, London and New York: Methuen.

Reason, J. T. (1982) 'Sensory processes', in Ann Taylor *et al.* (eds) *Introducing Psychology*, Harmondsworth, Mx: Penguin, pp. 218–52.

Reid, Louis Arnaud (1969) *Meaning in the Arts*, London: Allen & Unwin.

Richards, I. A. (1965) *The Philosophy of Rhetoric*, New York: Oxford University Press.

Ricoeur, Paul (1966) *Freedom and Nature: The Voluntary and the Involuntary*, trans. Erazim V. Kohak, Chicago, IL: Northwestern University Press.

Sartre, Jean-Paul (1956) *Being and Nothingness: A Phenomenological Essay on Ontology*, trans and intro. Hazel E. Barnes, New York: Washington Square Press.

Sheets-Johnstone, Maxine (1979) *The Phenomenology of Dance*, 2nd edn, London: Dance Books.

Sheets-Johnstone, Maxine (1984) 'Phenomenology as a way of illuminating dance', in Maxine Sheets-Johnstone (ed.) *Illuminating Dance: Philosophical Explorations*, London: Associated University Presses, pp. 124–45.

Sherrington, Charles S. (1973 [1906]) *The Integrative Action of the Nervous System*, New York: Arno Press.

Smith, Nancy Stark (1982) 'Dance in translation: the hieroglyphs', *Contact Quarterly* VII(2): 43–6.

Sparshott, Francis (1984) 'The dancing body: divisions on a Sartrian ground', in Maxine Sheets-Johnstone (ed.) *Illuminating Dance: Philosophical Explorations*, London: Associated University Presses, pp. 188–202.

States, Bert O. (1992) 'The phenomenological attitude', in Janelle G. Reinelt, Joseph R. Roach and Enoch Brater (eds) *Critical Theory and Performance*, Ann Arbor: University of Michigan Press, pp. 369–79.

Vesey, G. and Foulkes, P. (1990) *Collins Dictionary of Philosophy*, Glasgow: HarperCollins.

Youngerman, Suzanne (1984) 'Movement notation systems as conceptual frameworks: the Laban system', in Maxine Sheets-Johnstone (ed.) *Illuminating Dance: Philosophical Explorations*, London: Associated University Presses, pp. 101–23.

THE VOICE IN THE GARDEN SHED

Another day of stepping out this city, on my map once, years ago, there had been a stylized sheep framed in an oval and edged with blue, that was in the top right hand corner, sans serif type set underneath the image of the sheep said GOLDEN FLEECE, like the sheep that was printed red on yellow, what appeared to be graphic-ized sword blades radiated from this flock-ram logo, indicating the four points of the compass, the needle point of north crossed the

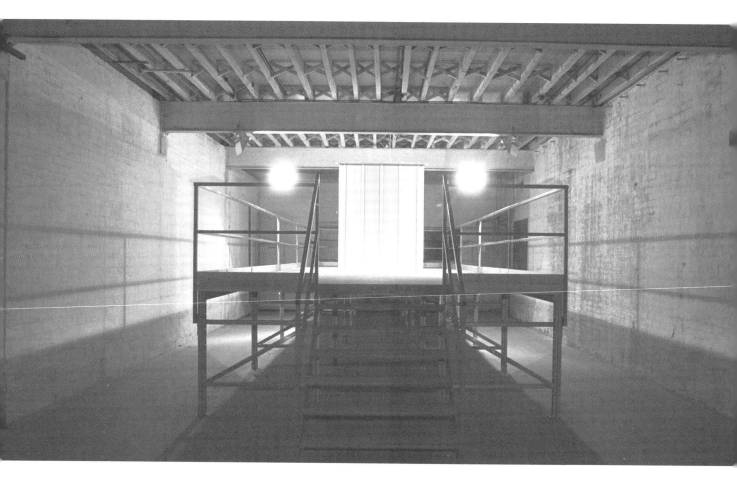

Torrens River - a meandering blue ribbon - at the junction of Walkerville Terrace and Stephen Road, a location on the map which I know well, a familiar location, part of my history in the city, this city, my city, this flesh rigid with fear, smelling sour with it, excrement, saps leaking, sphincters in spasm, this city is a map of myself, no, sorry, it is not a map of myself but a diagrammatic representation of me with the ribbon of blue, the Torrens, defining a contour across my face as viewed from the top, looking down upon my cranium, Montefiore Road, King William Road, and Frome Road, these connectors wire and plumb my head to my body so that thrilling shocks leaping the synapse

kick into life a cortex out of which leak juices too complex in their chemistry to emulate even though Wellington Square

is a repository for souvenirs, for this gas of intoxication which brings to a mechanistic corpse stalking interlocking

grids down the wiring and plumbing of Frome and Montefiore and King William, signals to let the body know it is alive

and thumbs tingle at the tips where just so much as the prick of a needle is too much to bear let alone if a splinter

should slither up under the nail of a probing finger while mind-body... which is walking, measuring city blocks from

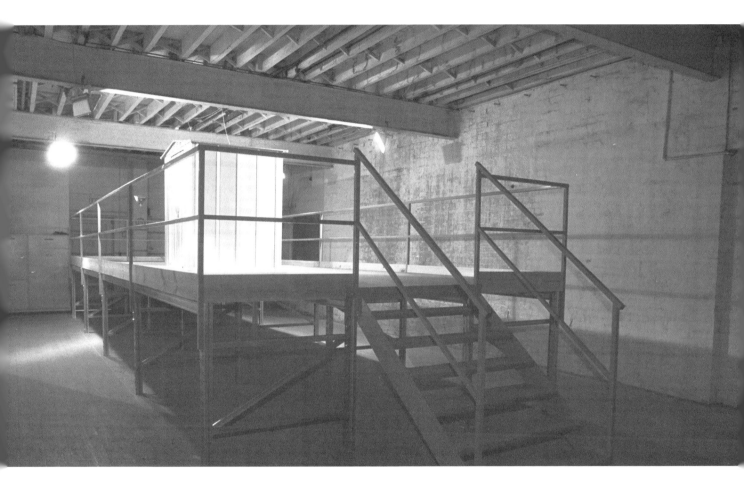

corner to corner, one foot in front of another, toe to heel, toe to heel to toe to heel, one foot at a time so that I travel

one thousand nine hundred and seventy-two feet on Carrington towards East Terrace where I might, except that

conscience carries me back to the University Bridge for I have done business there, my act dissected by shadows

hard on grass and within hearing of lions pissing out the corners of their territories (bitter salt sweat, the sweetness of

smeared faeces) measuring, step by step, a solitary circumnavigation of the globe of my head which has, if on my

map you follow Melbourne Street from between the West and South points of the GOLDEN FLEECE compass - that mildewed and silverfish-eaten long-gone map of mine - and turn off where streets are coloured the pink of mucus

membranes, so lubricous, so elastic that, and scented too because the essences are flowing out of glands - the brain

is a gland, North Adelaide a gland, Elizabeth too, and the River Torrens a drain transporting suburban poisons from

Athelstone and Thorndon Park, Klemzig, Gaza, Vale Park and Gilberton - out of the glands of my head, from my brain,

the pituitary, cortex, scattered cancer-vulnerable lymphs, a perverse pineal yearning for un-light under bridges so

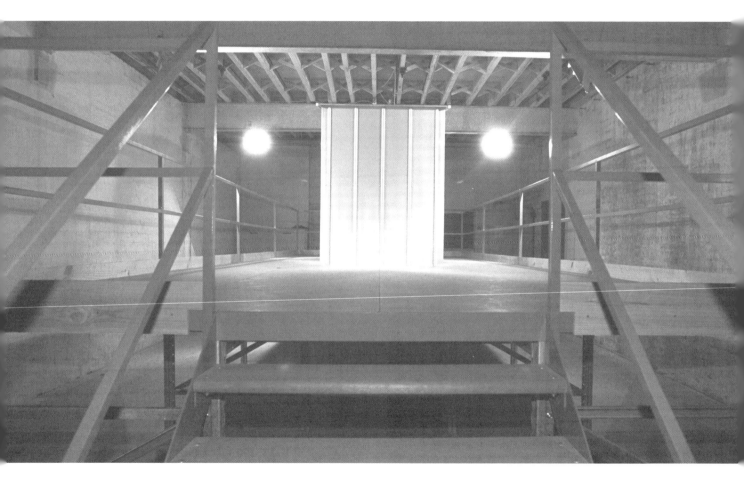

close to where the angry leopard, where the drip drip dripping juices flow down those drains which are Frome and

Montefiore and King William to infect with wonder, with undeniable itching arrogance, the five squares, Light and

Hindmarsh and Hurtle and Whitmore and Victoria, because my head is tilted forward and I am looking down, gazing

across the contour of my cheeks and nose as drawn by the cartographer, checking the far bank of the Torrens River,

that drain, that blue ribbon, that riband, that ribband, that blood soaked gauze, and because I demand the symmetry

of at least pain centred between being in the state of what I like to think of as pre-sensation - I am communicating with Victoria Square - in such a state that everything nature has put together in forming the entire corpse is a victim of the head, and waits, from the banal moment sliding in a sack of slime out of the belly of some near-spent organism, nothing but sensation which must - once it unstops the faucets and lets drip drip drip drip the precious essences, the juices of life discovery, Light discovery, from Frome and through King William, do not forget Hurtle and the others, my head is in Wellington Square where I have as history the dried parts which might have wasted if left attached as

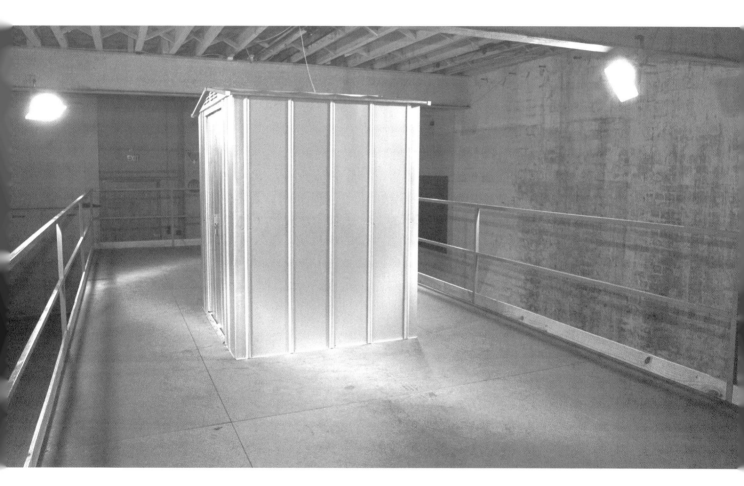

love tools to fools who couldn't know that where my head is tilted forwards and I gaze past the contour, eyebeams lasering across the Torrens River which is so beautifully alive with the vermin plastics and rubbers and foils drifting under the University Bridge from beneath which I have heard the jackal and the hyena and the aardvark snort, yap, snarl, call to the moon for some lead on which to build a plan of escape because I am wandering soon down King William to visit the so carefully laid out squares of my corpse and I am feeling the juices out of the gland inside my skull drip drip drip, snip snip snip, one foot placed in front of another foot, I am counting my way in search of souvenirs *of this grid which I am walking, this trip I am talking and taking through my own body, my head, my-God-created-self,*

trickling through the mechanics of what I am not, but appear to be if viewed as a silverfish-eaten chart foxed randomly

with brown spots, a chart which neither knows the delivery of terror nor the discreet slurping of semen as razor cuts

and this young and beautiful head comes awake to sensation precisely at the moment it is passing to the other side

of that same order of sensation, through an ecstasy of pain which was the salvation of us all through Jesus... mouth

suck at plastic and there is misting so that the outlines of this GOLDEN FLEECE chart, the map of a million feet

measured, retained in memory, has a sheep-red on yellow-in the top right hand corner and the points of the compass

as graphic-ized sword blades the tips of which stab into my consciousness where Robe Terrace is transformed into

Park Terrace beyond the intersection of Northcote and Walkerville Terraces and North is located where I have brought

sweet relief from the non-sensation swirling and cork-screwing into the vortex of my own mysterious chemistry which

comes from light and dazzles me even under the bridge or diving among ducks and swans and detritus close to where

caged panthers and moth-eaten wolves territorially piss, marking more than mere space but also and more importantly

the pace of the city and the suburbs and a hundred thousand million billion steps around the corners of rotating city

squares when closing in on Victoria and Hurtle and Whitmore and Hindmarsh and Light and Wellington.

In the Midst of Many: the Butcher, his Lover, her Husband, and the Hit Man

Linda Marie Walker

Like love . . . [a delicate and precise awareness of one's spatial relationships to the world] flourishes best on the very edge of loss of identity, of merging with the object; it is a dangerous leaning-over the brink of the blissfully all-dissolving oceanic, or of the seasick existential shudders. A cliff-edge experience.

(Robinson 1996: 105)

I wrote to a friend in Wyoming about this essay.

He wrote back: 'If I ever wrote about dance I would begin, "I am surrounded by unending space . . . and I am afraid" .'

I replied: 'I like how you would begin, I might use that. Why would you be afraid, I wonder. Is it the space, is it the body moving, being graceful or clumsy. Is it the body entering that space, worried about what it is, space I mean. Tell me.'

He: 'I think fear is the natural reaction if we stop to comprehend our place in the universe. Fear is close to awe, isn't it?' (from an email correspondence with Don White, 1997).

Today I received another type of letter. It said 'NO', and 'Why doesn't she use the fictive mode'. Or something like that, I tore it up. And this gesture (of anguish) now leaves me without the very thing, the exact words, that tormented me. I mean, I had written fiction, not ficto-criticism (as it was called in the letter), not essay, not thesis: 'writing'. I wanted to write music. I wrote the 'NO' text as a set of movements (perhaps 'steps'). Like a CD has songs (say, Nick Cave's 'The Boatman's Call'), or (more likely) like a set of country songs (say, the

Dead Ringer Band's 'Living in the Circle').

To summarize, 'NO' might have meant:

1 she moves (steps) across the surface, mapping this and that,
2 then, she doesn't 'develop' this and that.

Anyway . . . I am compelled to show my hand, to tell you this: this, this writing, is dancing; or, I imagine it as dance, as troubled limbs, repetitious steps; dance by small moves, called shiver, shudder, stagger, stumble. It's the heart constricted, it's tingles down the arms, it's breath sucked deep, it's panic, dying. It's the long drive to the hospital, in the early hours.

This is an extract from the 'NO' text:

I've been called a stranger. I've been thrown out of the lover's bed for being 'a foreigner', for having no language, for not speaking the language of the place where I am (was). And, me, who always thought the body spoke, knows now that language is expected for love, that sound is the wanted body. That I am nothing, no-woman, 'impossible' (this is impossible, said the lover, almost in 'my' language), in other words, when silent.

Performance Research 3(2), pp.59-66 © Routledge 1998

So, I will pretend to write this in silence.
There is no silence, the voice of the lover was loud.
I've been taught a lesson, I'm listening.

This piece (peace) of ('NO') writing is called *Ashtray Melancholy, short stories for Rafael*. It's about, or for, autobiography, it is autobiographical, about what happens (in the) everyday, about the awkward and awful and sodden and silly li/oved hours, and it's about when (or that) I rang Rafael from the telephone box near the church with the blue dome and spoke to his mother in his language, a little speech I had prepared on my way there, so that she might tell me if he was home, if he would come out and talk to me (walk with me), immediately. It's about that loneliness, and that friendship, and that gamble. It's about the whisky and gin we drank, and stayed sober. And it's about him saying to me: write. And me being overwhelmed by that word ('it' could have been 'play' instead, for instance), merely because he said it, because I heard it, and it seemed to mean something

I start; I start with the embarrassment of close-writing. And you, the reader, will fathom* the lover; the sadness of being the stranger is pervasive.

Here, the break, (write to me? he wrote), (or, I break the here), because I pause (write), to mention Mata Hari; they shot her, the military: it will be easy to forget that she is 'a break', that she is inside that break (suddenly, with her eyes open, she dropped to the ground, dead). She will fade away now and then – she's fading away, right now – in that drift (state) between awake and asleep. She will remain though, regardless (whether you or I remember) . . . and this is where the exchange, the substitution of 'break' for 'interval' begins . . . it just takes a while . . . continued.[†]

There are no new 'insights' here, 'here' is a text, not critical, not expository: a voice: 'I'd like to say . . .' Imagine, I write. Then cross it out. I write it

* 'Fathom: to *fathom*, originally "to embrace", deriving from Old English *faethmian*, to embrace, itself from OE *faethm*, the embracing arms, hence the full, straight stretch of both arms, hence the measure fathom (six feet) . . . akin to Old Saxon and *fathmos*, the outstretched arms . . . and can be compared to the Latin *patere*, to lie open, and *pandere*, to lay open' (Partridge 1982: 203).

again: imagine. I forget though what I was going to 'imagine' . . . and the word sits there, sullen.

This writing is (I imagine) something which parallels dance/performance. This crossing-out and retracing, this tearing-up and rejoining. I'm unsure. It's not a denial of outsides: hesitations, suggestions, conversations, reservations. The 'NO'. It's a speaking of it, a putting in circulation, despite anger (and shame).

The body shakes (following shiver and shudder) at the infinite cracks and crevasses by which speech and movement are thwarted. The body demands sound and touch, insists on being personal, being in the community. It walks down the ugly street, along the jetty (with the boys and girls who shout, shove, and give each other sly signs) and back again. It's a wisp of stuff, no more, no less.

I recall Saburo Teshigawara and Karas's dance-work in London (LIFT97) titled *I Was Real – Documents*. It was a work of repetition, like breathing is. Teshigawara said it was about air. It seemed to come from the inside, from the lungs or the stomach or the liver, and to be ordinarily threatening. I wrote this (June):

[it] is composed the way music is, as discrete movements, that sometimes have obvious passages between, and sometimes abruptly end, so that two pieces just join. One has to watch as one listens, remembering that one plays a piece of music again and again. And that repetition is a generous act (the heart beats). It gives the chance to see again, like sports replays do, like reading a novel for the fifth time does. Repetition makes room, pushes out

[†] Mata Hari was born on 7 August 1876 in Leeuwarden, a city in the north of Holland. As a girl she wore flamboyant clothes. 'One summer she wore a yellow and red striped dress, another time she came to school in red velvet, whirling and turning in front of her classmates, who were greatly impressed' (Waagenaar 1964: 20). 'While most girls of her age were dressed in demure, rather prim dresses, she wore flamboyant clothes (preferably in reds and yellows)' (Ostrovsky 1989: 13). From all that I have read of her, this I remember: a red dress. Something is how it begins. And, too, one will go on and on with what is near, at hand. The sense that cites the strange rising from the rundown buildings and parks is old, left over. The red dress is left over. Is quiet and heavy. Hardly worth mentioning. Setting a call to ugliness and terror, to come, one supposes, and to tiredness and time, to come, too. Terror in a minor key, a blue coating on the tongue, a few sounds of alien dread. To be never at home. (Walker, in Hoskin 1994: 11)

borders, creates the plaza, the plateau, where one gathers
with the crowd. Repetition is a relentless and resistant
way of 'speaking'. It's a force. Calling is repetition.
Although only one of Teshigawara's 'documents' uses the
'real' calling voice, the idea of calling seemed central to
each of the others. The call is bare, honest, imperfect.
When it happens there is no getting around it, and
nowhere else to be.

(http://www.rtimearts.com/~opencity/)

Also, perhaps, the call comes, often/always,
when one is alone. One calls alone, because one is
alone. This might mean, though, when in the midst
of many.

Today I watched a video sent to me by a friend
overseas. It was of two birthday parties; I briefly
saw myself at one. I saw the past, the past of me and
of them. And as I watched, I saw (constant, relentless, beautiful) movement. The bodies always in
some degree of motion, passing, reaching, smiling,
talking, eating, drinking. And a lot of blur, the
camera trying to focus. I watched these people
embrace, kiss, smoke, dance, sing, laugh. I watched
them being 'alive'. But more, I was given a dream,
they dreamed themselves toward me, because what
they gave was long over, and I was lost in pathos.
Yet, at the point of 'loss', I was sure, doubtless, that
'that' was all there was, for me. And 'that' was what
I could mention, exactly as if I had watched any
'performance'. That
attending the past is
crucial, and is a 'driven'
and delayed event.*

*See, for example, Roland Barthes
(1981), Hélène Cixous and Mireille
Calle-Gruber (1997), Maurice Blanchot
(1981) and Clarice Lispector (1988).

And, this is the beauty of 'dance' (its past): and
just as I write it, it's suddenly over, 'without'
counsel, that is, as if I can't say this, because it's
'known': archived, coming from the body's archive,
from cells, pulses, wounds, organs; and from
screeching, bending, blinking, stretching; from
vomiting, spitting, coughing, sneezing, shitting,
pissing, gasping; from pain, joy, love, hate. From
the daily doing of life. From jokes and clichés, from
'art' and 'soap', from tragedy and ecstasy. From
arriving and departing. There's no escape.

It's a strange idea, being a body, a space, a time.

And being, because a body, finite. Being finite,
finally. Surely this makes the body stall, startled.

I'm not sure; perhaps what situates, reveals, me
most is misreadings of comings-and-goings, their
fleeting possibilities. And what happens to 'one', to
one's body during those events; how does one 'say'
their (the events') consuming trauma. And this
drops from a great height: trauma.

There is trauma. All country music is about
trauma. Country music might be the music closest
to dance, to the restless body. It's music that doesn't
'mean' to dance, means to weep instead.

When I begin to write, it always starts from something
unexplained, mysterious and concrete . . . right away it
takes the poetic path. That is to say that it goes through
scenes, moments, illustrations lived by myself or by
others, and like all that belongs to the current of life, it
crosses very many zones of our histories. I seize these
moments still trembling, moist, creased, disfigured, stam-
mering.

(Cixous and Calle-Gruber 1997: 43)

This is the beginning, only . . . coming to, going
from, the place/region
where I should have
begun.†

† I ended a text this way: 'An
advent(ure) was underway, an essay, a
book of phrases from her time as
"Victoire", and something else, a
register of registers: "an 'it'", a space
half-entered" (Bataille 1991: 112). So
she writes herself something to
read (Hoskin 1994: 11)'.

The end of the
shiver, or stammer, the
last contraction, then
quiet. (I remember this
about *I Was Real – Documents*: we saw the end of
'events' – the left (over) air; ends seem dreadful,
last paroxysms that twist, contort and exhaust one's
desire. The question arises: can the body survive
these, which are so intense, absolute and possessed,
that as one gazes out from them, the world is
another place altogether. And no amount of excited
description will convey this: one mourns (for)
trauma. And thank god for mourning; the world, at
last, changed.)

I'm not sure.
    I'm exactly not sure, I mean.
    Take a step, step, step by, step by step.
    I step in time, unsteadily often, now: I go places.

Sometimes I dance, step-dance.

Trouble is, I probably write by stepping. Step-writing.

Step, see 'stamp' (which follows 'stammer' in Partridge's *Origins*): coming from the Old Norse word *stappa*, meaning to pound or stamp, and compare with the Old English word *steppan*, meaning to step, and with the German word *Stapfe*, meaning a footstep.

Perhaps then footstep-writing. Or, writing with the foot. Or, writing with my foot in my mouth. Or, writing with two left feet. Tripping, easily. Falling.

Leaving home by foot, returning home by foot. Passing over, across the earth. Mapping space and place by touch, by the touch of the foot.

I could be mapping something here, too, creeping up on death even, I'm not sure. I'm trying to-step, to make-steps, towards writing, this writing, which comes word by word: the day is warm, there is a slight sea breeze, the phone rings: untangle legs, rise from chair, stand, turn, walk, dodge armchair, pick up receiver: hello. Two syllables: hell-o. And someone speaks to me.

Now I'll stop writing for awhile, go outside, pick beans, water a geranium, procrastinate (in other words).

Recently I was walking through sandhills near where a body had been found. And, so the story goes, there's another yet to surface. (The story's quite a good one as it might be that the town has eaten it – the missing body/person, and that's food for thought.) Anyway, I wondered about dancing murder, or as it came to me (then), about writing murder into dance (what could this writing look like, what could writing look like as murder-movement-notation).

Bernard Tschumi choreographs music into architecture, maps architecture as event, space, motion, along time lines (moments, intervals, sequences) which are combinative; that is, layered, compressed, expanded, isolated. And this so as *not* to represent or mime, but 'to underline the fact that

perhaps all architecture, rather than being about functional standards, is about love and death' (Tschumi 1994: xxviii).

Map: I've taken a liberty with this word. Yes, as it's defined: a 'representation' of a portion of the earth's surface. Impossible.

> We could not use or even bear to look at a map that was not mostly blank. This emptiness is to be filled in with our own imagined presence, for a map is the representation, simultaneously, of a range of possible spatial relations between the map-user and a part of the world.
>
> (Robinson 1996: 106)*

* 'I prefer the step [to roots] – indefinitely repeatable and variable – as a metaphor of one's relationship to a place' (Robinson 1996: 213).

Going on, taking another step, cutting to this:

> They found the Transcripts by accident. Just one little tap and the wall split open, revealing a life-time's worth of metropolitan pleasures – pleasures that they had no intention of giving up. So when she threatened to run and tell the authorities, they had no alternative but to stop her. And that's when the second accident occurred – the accident of murder. . . . They had to get out of the Park quick. But one was tracked, by enemies he didn't know – and didn't even see – until it was too late.
>
> (Tschumi 1994: 14)

The architectural drawings (the movement-notations) which follow this scenario (and the other three) are of

> spatial effects: the movement of bodies in space . . . as if the dancer had been 'carving space out of a pliable substance'; or the reverse, shaping continuous volumes, as if a whole movement had been literally solidified, 'frozen' into a permanent and massive vector.
>
> (Tschumi 1994: 10)

To return to the sandhills and the body: how can the landscape of the murder, a landscape familiar to me (my home town), be talked about now, how does one walk in it now; the denseness of the scrub might have hidden the body for ages if the murderers had been more 'professional'. And this: at any moment we might locate (or smell: 'A strong odour alerted police to the presence of the body') the missing one.* One's steps are more acute, more potentially potent, perhaps. This seems to indicate a death-dance, steps speaking violence. Is speech dance, are syllables steps? For example, the stammer: ohhh III lllllloooovvee the ssilent ssspace offf waaaiting. The story of murder is stammered, people interjecting, correcting, adding. It's about a 'butcher'. It's about a butcher, his lover, her husband, and a hit man. Bluey (and Bluey might be imagined), the hit man, is missing.†

* *The Southern Eastern Times*, Millicent, Monday 27 June 1994: cover. Also, somewhere in *Beloved* Toni Morrison wrote: 'You know as well as I do that people who die bad don't stay in the ground.'

† "There was also a plan to get 'Bluey' to kill [Mr A] for $500 but he was a figment of the imagination of [Mr L]," said Mr Rice (counsel for [Mrs A']' (*The South Eastern Times*, n.d.).

Stepping is a way of moving over the surface, rambling, mooching, prowling, drifting, straying, sneaking, strolling, limping, strutting, tracking. Stepping paces-out space. We step through space, measuring ourselves from things, by things, and from and by motion (birds, cars, animals, clouds, trees): we pass, and are passed.

> We are spatial entities – which is even more basic than being material entities, subject to the laws of gravity. The barest of bones of the relationship between an individual and the world are geometrical; on the landscape scale, topographical. Our physical existence is at all times wrapped in the web of directions and distances that constitutes our space. Space, inescapable and all-sustaining Space, is our unrecognized god.
>
> (Robinson 1996: 104–5)

I wonder how murder begins, what prompts the first thought, and how that thought feels: scary, alarming, exhilarating. Here's a room. It's a room upstairs, a bar. There are three people. I cut now, in this writing, from a 'scene' of stepping (and murder) to a 'scene' of sitting (and thinking):

> 'Could you tell me once more,' said the man. 'It's the sound of the wind,' said the woman.
>
> The man kept his hands spread wide on his thighs. She added nothing, looking at him.
>
> 'And what is it that sounds like the wind,' he said. 'Nothing at all, but the very end, the light too,' she said.

The day was near turning dusk, although the warmth remained.

'You don't know then,' he said, right before her, a steady stare.

She wanted to say something. He was waiting for an exclamation, a few words of panic even. But she was thinking, being careful perhaps, her eyes wide. Someone nearby stood up and walked away.

'Eva,' he said, 'you are not the only one here.'

She took a long breath. Across the room a child, a man really, looked away, he'd been watching her, and the gold light of the sunset. He liked her, her cheeks high and brown, her white eyes.

'I have said it before, I've said it thousands of times, thousands and thousands, and you never remember, that is true as I am here,' he said.

The woman couldn't think of a thing to say, as he was right. She looked at the boy-man as if he was a flame on the horizon. She began to mumble under her breath.

'Here,' she said, 'always here.'
'You,' he said, 'won't talk in the glare, that's a fact, it's no more than that.'

She looked at the boy again, at all of him, especially his head, and she was cold and bare towards him.‡

‡ An extract from an unpublished text: 'The stories of Eva Beatrice' (novel) or 'Script for the Theatre of No/thing'.

In the room steps (small moves) take place in stillness and in voice. As if each person is slowly moving toward, or away from, the other, while being physically fixed. The literal stepping is over, they arrived (perhaps by slow sad or fast firm steps). Has one of these, or all, had a murder-thought? Has murder crossed their minds, discreetly, almost imperceptively, or have they dwelt on it, over coffee or during a long night?

There is an interval in stepping: the curved space the foot makes between leaving the ground and returning to it. The interval, a space, is the passage of to-step. To-step is to-move through the air. And in the room the trio make steps with air (voice). Somewhere else I called this 'break', not 'interval'. Interval has a different spatial tone and ambience from 'break', it acknowledges the continuum, the relation, of all 'events', of all mediums. The interval is a space within which speaking comes about: a be-speaking, be-spoken, place. It was wild, despairing ('break'), now it is (be-coming) calm, gentle, pleasurable ('interval'). Interval-speaking can afford more time, and less. As if one doesn't, anymore, have to 'speak' of the 'break' as actual. And in speaking 'interval' one doesn't, anymore, have to actually speak it, it seems already said, to be itself (interval) an interval (a space between), a pause (an interval in-interval): the intermezzo: the intervening space . . .

Barthes, writing of the music of Schumann:

> The intermezzo . . . has as its function not to distract but to displace: like a vigilant sauce chef, it keeps the discourse from 'setting', from thickening, from spreading, from returning obediently into the culture of *development* [my emphasis]; it is this renewed act (as every speech-act is renewed) by which the body stirs and disturbs the hum of artistic speech. At the limit, there are only intermezzi: *what interrupts is in its turn interrupted* [my emphasis], and this begins all over again. One might say that the inter-mezzo is *epic* (with the meaning Brecht gave this word . . .'
>
> (Barthes 1991: 300)*

* I'm sure that Miles Davis's *In A Silent Way* is one epic intermezzo.

. . . and interval is poorer, more scant, than break. Being in the interval is forever (as a momentary sensation: lost-for-words, glued-to-the-spot, for instance). It is speaking as it is spoken, and writing as it is written, which interferes with, and gives us, the aloneness of living intervally.

> We are in the world thanks to this scant being [the interval]. And it's the scant being of our being – or our sharing – that calls for so much speaking. Little being = lots of speaking, for you never get done designating the interval. You never finish speaking – which explains the ever so singular, obstinate murmur of every variety of literature (although everything has already been said, if you will, for a long time now). But one speaks so that the abundance of

speech – every instant, or as often as possible – lets the scanty being, our existence, show through.

(Nancy and Smock 1993: 318)

Slowly stepping back(wards) to the room . . . just letting you know (Tawa and Walker 1997).[†]

> My relationship with a friend has become so simple and free that I often telephone her and, when she picks up the receiver, I explain I am not in the mood for conversa-tion. So I say goodbye, replace the receiver and occupy myself with something else.
>
> (Lispector 1992: 328)

[†] I think of 'table' (prompted by the tables in 'the room'). Of the table on which one writes, and on which one imagines one would like to write, the table by the window looking out onto the 'scene'. I have been starting this writing, kicking it into the next stage, and going too fast, then too slow, staging it by starting over, yet a little further on, as if not 'at home' – and wanting to be, and wanting there to be a 'home', a place to stay. I'm telling you of a world which is not yours. I wonder about the everyday of being by oneself, in community, in the very country of one's birth. But then to shift inside that country, to move from the 'country' to the 'city'; to be always 'country' at heart and 'city' at heart, at once. To be with three hearts, to be tricrotic: to have three undulations for each beat of the heart. The undulations being with, and passing, each other, strangers to one another: a tricrotous being. (Fragments of *In the Midst of Many*, like the one above, are drawn from a paper written collaboratively with Michael Tawa, 1997.)

This freedom seems a breath away from 'You never finish speaking'. The need to say 'I don't feel like speaking', and 'I want to speak that to you'. The calling toward someone, the calm which greets the other's answer (hello) then lets you go, and doesn't want more than your going-away, your being-absent, even as you speak. It's a type of migrating, of having to leave and not leaving until the friend is told; of turning about, (un)winding, and yet connecting to where one knows one is, and wanted. The sense of loss that being alone clarifies, while knowing one can 'call' and say, 'I am going now'. As there is no release from that going-away. A goodbye, which promises return, and which nourishes the one who gets on with 'something else'. This leaving is an on-loan leaving, a leaving done again and again. A leaving; a return: tomorrow, next week, next year. Sooner or later the migrant returns (home, and is always returning in speech, longing, writing, memory), leaves by (stepping, intervally) 'calling'. And there is terror too, the violence (murder) of not being able (at the last moment) to do this calling (a summoning of help, courage), of having been ripped-away, of not then having the freedom 'to occupy myself with something else'. This freedom depends on the freedom to call, to speak: the freedom of the heart to not-break, to 'interval' instead.

Remember, a body is still (perhaps) in the sandhills (near the Bevilaqua Ford Bridge), or eaten (is still being eaten).*

Back in the room:

The man raised his voice slightly, hardly at all. 'Look at me,' he said.

She was a little shaken. He folded his arms, he'd been caught out. The music began, a radio close by, off the station, a haze of hiss, but not disturbing, behind a song she'd heard often lately. The boy was listening too. And he was looking at her sometimes, briefly. He was comfortable, his hands lightly on the table, smooth and soft, creamy vegetable things.

'It's not an easy decision,' she said, half-heartedly, more to herself than him, although for sure he heard. The boy turned, shifted his body, facing her. I could touch you, she thought, he was making her see him as a target, as a moving vehicle. He laced his fingers on the table.

'Let's pretend then that neither of us wants to talk,'

*A map of the area where the body was found appeared in the local paper, the spot was marked with an "X". In a later story, in the same paper, of proceedings at day four of the trial Mrs M, a crown witness (who had earlier pleaded guilty to the charge of administering a noxious substance to Mr A (the body), and who had been granted immunity from prosecution in return for giving evidence against the accused, Mr L and Mrs A) was asked about Bluey, the hit man, still missing. She said Mr L knew Bluey from Vietnam. ' "[Mr L] got [Mr A] to go to a house in Olive Street to fix up a camper on his four wheel drive. [Mr A] was going to be lured into a pit-cellar in the garage and 'Bluey' was going to be there to kill him. [Mrs A] said she had $1,000 for 'Bluey'." [Mrs M] said that night (a Wednesday), she had been playing a game called "Greed" with [Mrs A] at the caravan park. "[Mrs A] became agitated and shocked and went white when [Mr A] walked in", said [Mrs M]. On the following Friday, [Mrs M] said she had been sitting in the carpark of a . . . supermarket with [Mrs A] in her vehicle. "[Mr L] came and saw us and said everything had gone wrong. He [Mr L] said while [Mr A] was still there (the Olive Street house), he went to the bedroom to talk to Bluey. When he got to the bedroom, he said that Bluey was on dope and he was demanding more and more money and that things didn't work out. [Mr A] went home and after . . . there had been an argument and [Mr L] had lost his temper and bashed Bluey and said he'd killed him," said [Mrs M]. The witness said that [Mr L] had told her that "Bluey" was in the pit in the garage at Olive Street. [Mrs M] said she went to the Olive Street house on the next day (a Saturday) and had used "Plush" carpet cleaner to make the stain lighter. "A bladder from a water bed was on the line and that was used to wrap the body in the pit. [Mr L] said that he buried 'Bluey' under a bridge".' (*The Southern Eastern Times*, Monday 13 February 1995, p. 4.)

he said, the man, 'one has to do what one is told, or the ship sinks.'

Silence, the sound only of the outside, a little traffic on the street, a few birds, what she called night-birds, and the scent of a vine, a definite greenness. And Spring, in its first glassy return, a faint tone in the ear.

The man said, 'Are you certain, am I to believe you are reluctant?'[†]

† Extract from an unpublished text: 'The Stories of Eva Beatrice' (novel) or 'Script for the Theatre of No/thing'.

I am not sure, exactly.

It seems that what I've written is merely one interval, one step.

I was intending to go a little further, two steps.

I began with the reply from a friend. He wrote: 'I would begin, "I am surrounded by unending space . . . and I am afraid".'

That's 'it' and 'is' (the present): unending space. The interval of unending space. And the ways of being in that, step by step.

I love the sandhills I've mentioned (and when I'm in them they seem eternal) and the treacherous coastline they shield; for me they help to counter – together with the murder(s), and all the other stories I know of them (I saw the eclipse of the sun there in the 1970s), and the way they make my body ache for days afterwards – the ideal of 'development'. They pile up, one upon the other, as worlds; overlapping, interweaving, polyrhythmic, sensations, events and materials, effecting (infecting) each other beyond any possible sustained narrative.

The totality of geometric relations between the individual and the world is more than infinitely dense, and even the mere set of directions from me to other things or places forms an uncountable continuum.

(Robinson 1996: 105)

Of course, back in the room life goes on.

And they, scanty beings, speak, hear, watch, so to live, so to continue their stepping, the making/writing of their continual interval with each other:

Through the square window she could see the tops of brown chimneys with their dull steel funnels. The boy too looked out the window, they were both distracted for a moment, hardly long enough to be counted as time, but a cut, a scratch, a hair crack. A first meeting, a rendezvous. Everywhere, all over the city chimneys just like these, were being watched, a low pleasure, for the sake of peace. The gold light was gone, the sky already a pale grey with last rays making a line across the wall behind her. Two small black birds flew above the chimneys, as big as cinders.

'Don't you see,' he said, 'the end of it cannot be just the sound of the wind.'

The two birds flew back and sat briefly on the edge of a gutter, bobbing up and down, balancing in the breeze.

She tried to think of another way of telling him how it seemed to her.

She did not wish him ill, but she was nervous of his focus on her, its suddenness too, as if thrown out as bait, and beyond her, and yet within proximity, and in all honesty (what's more) there was nowhere else she'd planned to be.

'What a disaster, what a fine mess,' he said.*

* ibid.

REFERENCES

Barthes, Roland (1981) *Camera Lucida: Reflection on Photography*, trans. Richard Howard, New York: Hill & Wang.

Barthes, Roland (1991) 'Rasch', in *The Responsibility of Forms: Critical Essays on Music, Art, and Representation*, trans. Richard Howard, Berkeley and Los Angeles: University of California Press.

Bataille, George (1991) *The Impossible*, trans. Robert Hurley, San Francisco: City Lights Books.

Blanchot, Maurice (1981) *The Madness of the Day*, trans. Lydia Davis, New York: Station Hill Press.

Cixous, Hélène and Calle-Gruber, Mireille (1997) *Rootprints, Memory and Life Writing*, trans. Eric Prenowitz, London and New York: Routledge.

Hoskin, Teri (ed.) (1994) *Lacuna*, Adelaide: Teri Hoskin.

Lispector, Clarice (1988) *The Passion According to G.H.*, trans. Ronald W. Sousa, Minneapolis: University of Minnesota Press.

Lispector, Clarice (1992) 'Freedom', in *Discovering the World*, trans. Giovanni Pontiero, London: Carcanet Press.

Nancy, Jean-Luc and Smock, Ann (1993) 'Speaking without being able to', in *The Birth to Presence*, trans. Brian Holmes *et al.*, Stanford, CA: Stanford University Press.

Ostrovsky, Erika (1989) *Eye of Dawn: The Rise and Fall of Mata Hari*, New York: Dorset Press.

Partridge, Eric (1982) *Origins: A Short Etymological Dictionary of Modern English*, London: Routledge & Kegan Paul.

Robinson, Tim (1996) 'On the Cultivation of the Compass Rose', in *Setting Foot on the Shores of the Connemara & Other Writings*, Dublin: The Lilliput Press.

Tawa, Michael and Walker, Linda M. (1997) 'Delinquent practices: drifting writing architecture', in Stephen Cairns and Philip Goadin (eds) *Building, Dwelling, Drifting, Migrancy and the Limits of Architecture: Papers from the 3rd 'Other Connections' Conference*, Melbourne: University of Melbourne.

Tschumi, Bernard (1994) *The Manhattan Transcripts*, London: Academy Editions.

Waagenaar, Sam (1964) *The Murder of Mata Hari*, London: Arthur Barker.

Punto di Fuga: an Afterword

Peter Stafford

Australia is the driest and flattest continent on the planet. In just over two hundred years it has been environmentally devastated – possibly beyond repair. This is the psychic residue of the colonial past. Once Australia was a distant resource, an exotic 'under-land' to be exploited and possibly explored; now its people have begun to examine the question of independence in earnest – coincidentally, at a time when public awareness of environmental chaos reaches a critical mass.

It is a disheartening paradox that a performer working in the most isolated city in the world should need to imagine the flight of birds (of the wilderness) in order to envisage a vantage point beyond the artificial enlightenment of Western technological culture. From those, and that, which is in dangerous retreat, the (still) wild birds and rare clear waters, I take heart. They are yet beyond technique and ratio . . .

As a writer and performer I am particularly concerned with the interface between text, performance and context or environment. The text that follows was written to accompany an exhibition/performance in March 1996 in Perth.* It imparts a series of metaphors that, following Gregory Bateson, are intended to work in unison to create patterns that connect across disparate space and time. Moreover, the text has a complementary aspect, in that it works with, and between, a series of images, sounds and gestures. Together, these suggest a possible way through the noise of postmodernity without negating it.

* *Punto di Fuga/Message Sticks*, at the Cullity Gallery, Perth, 17 February–1 March 1996; a performance by Peter Stafford and Felicity Bott, with sound by John Patterson, lighting/video by Graeme McLeod; dramaturgical assistance by Barry Laing.

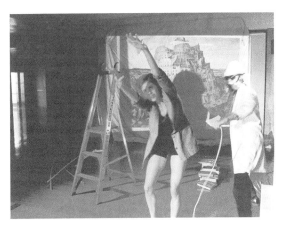

Punto di Fuga/Message Sticks, 1996: Felicity Bott, Peter Stafford

In parallel with the performance/exhibition the text provides connections, clues for audience members wanting to construct their own imaginative road through the network of signification that arises both within and without the performative space. All of the forty-odd paintings coupled to the forty-minute performance by myself and Felicity Bott create a series of imaginative associations which evoke a sense of metaphorical patternings. Ideally these connect across the gaps through a range of sites and temporalities.

Water and light intersperse the text and performance as metaphors that bind all being into a single web of global interdependence. Yet here in Australia, the light has taken on a cancerous aura and the water has become irrevocably polluted. A nation that actively seeks to become a new republic also stands virtually alone in refusing to undertake an internationally determined commitment to reduce greenhouse gas emissions.

At the beginning of the performance, a blind art gallery director stares into the open end of a nautilus

Performance Research 3(2), pp.67–74 © Routledge 1998

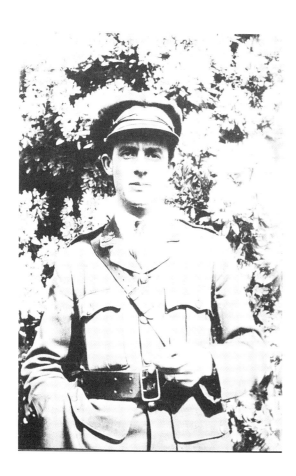

F/LIGHT MATTERS

> . . . Silently the birds
> Fly through us. O, I who long to grow,
> I look outside myself, and the tree inside me grows.
> (Rainer Maria Rilke, August 1914)

On the night that he died, I visited my grandfather. He had been left lying on a metal trolley awaiting amputation in a dimly lit hallway of the repatriation hospital. In a state of semi-waking, he was struggling to rip the web (net) of drips out of his body so that he could, as he said, 'be free' . . . but to do what? One of the few still living pilots from the First World War, what could he do? . . . Fly down the corridors, back through the years . . .

Since childhood I have been fascinated with things that fly – magic balloons, pelicans and aeroplanes, in that order. Aeroplanes are like arrows, tools that function at the behest of their pilots, and magic balloons do not exist for adults. Pelicans, however, lilt and swoop, honk and hover of their own volition. They are beasts of wilderness and desolation. Indeed, in the Old Testament they are associated with the 'plumbline of the void'. Yet, fickle as the history of 'man' and metaphors proves to be, pelicans were gradually transformed by human projection until they became, in the medieval bestiaries and for Dante and others following, a symbol of the love that Christ emanates for humanity.*

* Interestingly, decanters in alchemy, used for concocting who knows what, were called 'pelicans' and usually took the form of human testicles or breasts.

In the human mind, pelicans may embody such mythic resonances; however, they have no real relation to our purposes, other than our destruction of their nesting grounds, their homes. When they take flight pelicans move with a strange logic that befits the mystery that the ancients accorded them. Huge beasts of both water and ground, they take flight, unlike the aeroplane and its pilot, with no trajectory or end point in mind. Their trajectory, function, or purpose, is of a different order.

As a boy, I built glider planes from balsa wood sticks and covered them with lacquered paper. Aeroplanes are, metaphorically speaking, sticks . . .

shell whilst at the end of the piece he imagines himself as a child imitating a pelican. In this guise, he and a symbolic mother figure pass out of the performance space and plant a tree which has spent the duration of the three-week exhibition under an artificial hydroponic light. The text that follows was intended to open a space beyond the vanishing point, the *punto di fuga* – that abstract location where, in classical perspective, water and light cease to 'matter' in a qualitative sense. The writer-artist-performer knows that should an audience's members seek another layer of depths beyond those of the performative body or the representational image, they can further explore a relatively coherent series of patterns through the following text. Patterns discovered therein may connect in a mind beyond the darkness of the performance space long after the lights have gone down, the birds have flown and the tree has been planted . . .

tools for departure that care not for human projections. They are entirely the product of a rational attention to the laws of physics. Their message, to explore further the metaphoricity of the machine, is one of function. Like sophisticated arrows, they are pointed at some future-orientated destiny. Aeroplanes are the result of an experimental mode of observation which could calculate the gravitational effect of a man on the moon long prior to his actual arrival.

Yet, I somehow doubt that this man will ever arrive there again. The gravity of our problems right here, now, due to the fact of the 'matter' will probably resist his escape velocity.

Still, what does it matter? The world is a truly spectacular place, more so for human specialization and the subsequent mystification of technological mediation. We may wonder at the apparent brilliance of human 'progress' – whilst knowing very little about what has actually been discovered along the relentless path toward absolute technological control of the natural world.

And what of the ghosts that shadow these dreams of technological mastery over the primitive, the animal, the 'base' matter in us? Those who departed through the vanishing point of would-be technical utopias? The witches, the insane, hysterics, Frankenstein's monsters, replicants, anorexics, mass murderers, aliens, 'primitives', theoretical physicists, mystics and even, occasionally, 'artists'. . . . Are these dark 'others' symptomatic of the resistance of matter to be 'accelerated'?

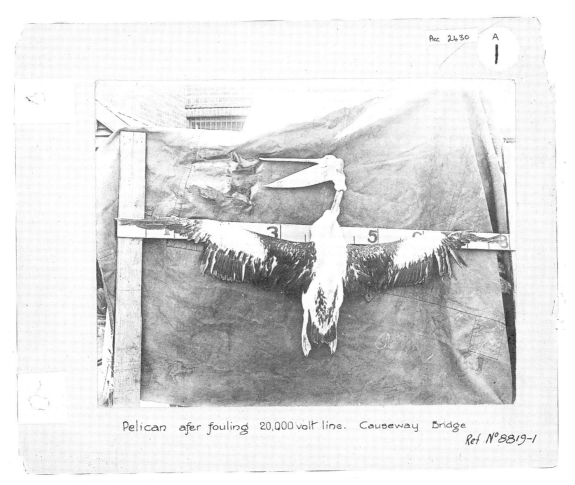

Pelican afer fouling 20,000 volt line. Causeway Bridge
Ref Nº 8819-1

Photo: Photographer unknown, 1930

Have they refused to be re/placed into the homogenous space of mathematicized Econoscience? . . . In other words, 'will they not be en'light'ened?'

Australian Aboriginals use wooden message sticks to signify a certain kind of presence. The sticks are not really tools but, literally, metaphors which have no meaning without a messenger or outside a particular context. There is nothing 'written' on them. There is no wording, they are a gesture of communication, often a rite of passage or an amplification of a declaration of intent. It is clearly understood that the message is not *in* the stick but, rather, is articulated through its web of relations to a wider context.

My current performance is entitled *Message Sticks*. In it I use a range of tools or 'sticks' to look at

what happens when the faculty of metaphor is restricted to entirely practical purposes, to the modernizing task propounded by technological fundamentalism. In such instances, when the metaphor is taken literally the user of the stick enacts a reflex that is usually both unconscious and habitual. When exploring this situation in the performative context, the two performers are placed in a space between the reflexive determinacy of the 'script' or 'message' (stick) and the indeterminacy of the audience's reception, response and interaction.

Descartes believed that the reflex of the body (as he would 'think it') was 'mindless'. Yet, neither the stick nor the body is mindless, unless their relation becomes one of reflex. Reflex – the robot is the ultimate reflexive body – signifies the death of the imagination limited by an uncritical acceptance of ideological limits. We see the qualitative difference

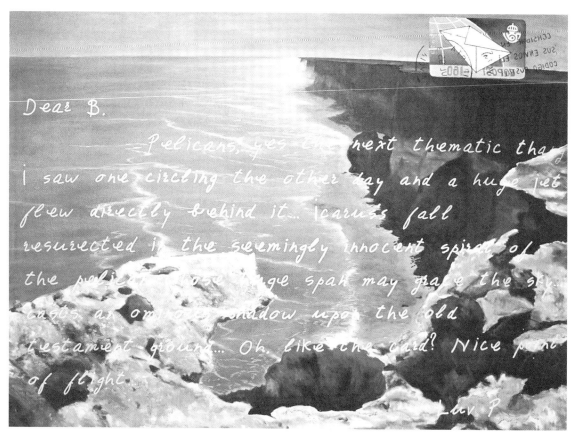

Punto di Fuga/Message Sticks, 1996

between reflex and imagination in Frankenstein's monster's retreat to the Arctic and the replicant's eventual rescue of his would-be 'exterminator' in *Blade Runner*.

In *Message Sticks* I have a spirit level, a shovel, a golf stick, a T-square, a blind stick and much more. . . . They are all mediated 'sticks' that *message* – some more immediate than others. It is the humble 'stick', the first tool, in its natural immediacy that has a perfect memory of the tree. The tree reaches deep into this earth and draws up water filtered through the ground. A stick is a dead tree without water exchange. It cannot breathe, it is literally alive but at a microcosmic level only visible through a light-processing machine. Modernity, however, advances the context within which we see water and trees.

As we dream of a departure, of an escape from the mortality that such technologies as the Pioneer 10 and our celluloid film shadows have already surpassed, so we continue to create new technologies for the flight from the place where matter is simply a given.

Yet, in all of this, it is the water and trees that *actually* depart. This 'desertion', in turn, approaches with the world-wide occurrence of encroaching deserts.

Matter is increasingly accelerated in 'convergence circuits', and converted into light. (The so-called enlightenment has its literal corollary in the exponential creation of those mutual quantities of light and entropy.) Just as we have complex systems of water dispersal, so we have personal matter converters – screens – that transform matter into light. With the Copernican revolution we become a fire planet, one of concentrated (focused) light and fire rather than one of water and dispersal. Through our various light converters powered by fire (from the burning of fossil fuels to the splitting of the atom), we literally make matter fly from its place – we depart(mentalize) the world and reconstruct it as light.

But how has this powerful reduction of the world into laser-like light enlightened us?

Most of my artworks and performances to date

have been framed by the irrational image of water as a kind of binding metaphor. Like the pelican, a water bird, it has been subject to human projections. Perhaps, because we ourselves are mostly constituted of water, we are apt to reconstitute its place and make-up in the scheme of things in much the same way as we reinvent our identities. And yet the infinite qualitative range of both identity and water is subject to the limits of our imaginative desires. Even as the artist/performer may attempt to rescue the identity from the normative forces of ideological consensus, so, too, might s/he strive to re-create the life of water, liquid matter, within the confines of modernity's mono-focus.

As the lines within the nautilus shell – which Icarus smashed to find the source of its sound – tell us, the moon was once far closer to the earth and consequently the planet must have been covered in water. Noah had to cut down trees to save us from

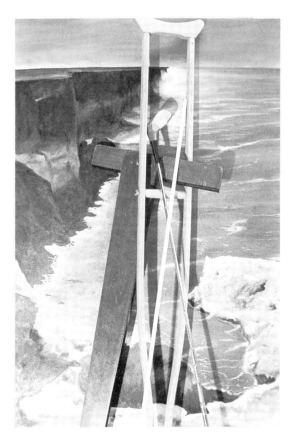

Punto di Fuga/Message Sticks, 1996

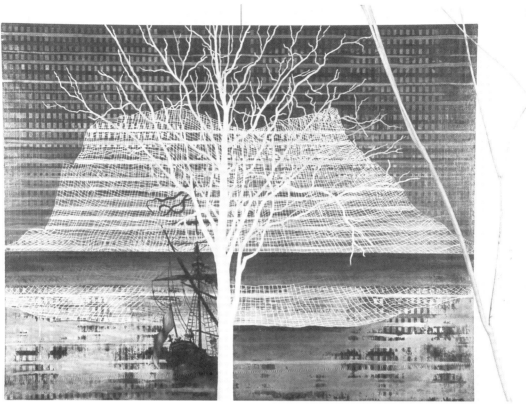

Punto di Fuga/Message Sticks, 1996

the flood (a fine argument for fundamentalist tree-fellers). Even as the fire of modernity smouldered into life, Leonardo was still depicting a world ending in torrential flooding. But to reiterate, modernity is the great 'context' shifter: it is the context. With modernity and the introduction of a way of seeing and acting upon the world from behind the window of technique, contexts are inevitably de-parted – relegated to a point beyond the vanishing point – or *punto di fuga*, the point of flight, as Alberti first named it.*

* See Robert Romanyshyn, *Technology as Dream and Symptom* (London: Routledge, 1989). I owe much of the above to Romanyshyn's prescient writing on technology as a 'symptomatic' vehicle for our dreams of departure – from the earthbound body.

The departure of the context beyond the horizon of human light projection means fewer trees, more sticks and deserts – more empiricist Noahs – and less clear water. The Moors cut down the oaks, the Lebanese the cedars, as great armies and places of worship arose and fell. The Spanish Armada and therefore the Spanish forests went to the bottom of the English Channel (as did much of Sherwood Forest), but not so the British sea captains who, having so advanced their usage of Dutch mapping techniques – made possible by the invention of linear perspective and the CVP – were able to beget our ascendants over here, who likewise proceeded to fell trees; meanwhile the desert advanced and the water muddied. (It is possible to measure the shift in rainfall after the construction of the rabbit-proof fence.)

So water, like the standardized countenance of reason and progress, is getting murkier. Modernity passes into Postmodernity as clarity – read 'focused vision' – burns the pages upon which have been written the rules that are to be applied, without heed of context. We have set fire to the playground and the resultant ashes are poisonous.

Never mind the oil wars, the coming water battles would turn both Noah and Leonardo in their graves (for they are not cremated in some hidden gas-fired furnace but lie still buried in the wet earth).

As a painter and garden owner, I waste and probably pollute my share of fresh water. We need trees but do we need more images? Which is more in need of the life of colour, the desert or the blank canvas? They are, perhaps, one and the same, signs of a desire for the fluid, for a need to reflect.

We are flooded with light-energized images and yet ever more fearful of water shortages.

Beuys might even have argued that we need less imagery and more trees – he certainly initiated the planting of a good many. The manipulator of light and matter, the artist/performer is a modern Faust aware of both his tradition as a history of bathos and of the continuing desire to colour the undifferentiated desert. It is a need to form an imaginative ground and, bathetic as it is, it will be at least for myself a turn to the blue. Blue for water, sky – the

flight of magic balloons, pelicans and balsa wood planes – transformation, depression, transition, the planet seen from space, and because Yves Klein at the height of his bathetic career said so.

In this current exhibition there is a lot of blueness mixed within fields of differentiation and non-differentiation, of material presences immanent but out of sight across fields that are, perhaps, in-sight. There is, as Leonardo says somewhere, the great thing of the being of nothing-ness. There is no point to this, only an orientation. The soul, as James Hillman reminds us, is not a thing but an orientation that is not a given.

Somewhere in a forest of blue there may be a point of flight, of departure, that leads beyond con-traction. The vanishing point flips over and expands again to reveal a cleavage in the visual crypt. Another way of seeing Alberti's *punto di fuga* is as an emanation point – of divine light. But it is not the banal 'project/ive' eye of the ideological God: that supreme authority, given vent via the reductive focus

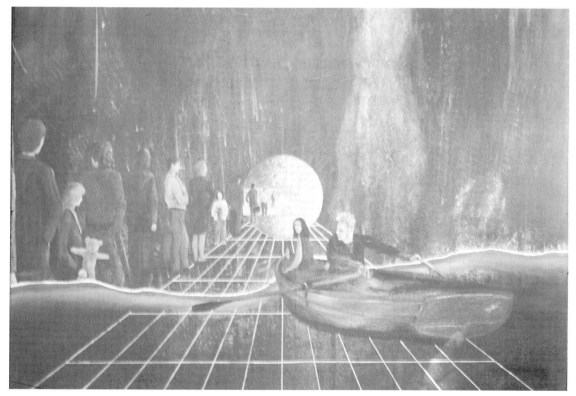

Punto di Fuga/Message Sticks, 1996

of modernity's future-obsessed vision that departs its context and explodes what (it) matters. It is of the dispersive, binding quality of water rather than the focused anatomizing power of fire and information. This is a qualitative light beyond all quantitative explanation. One either intuits it or not. It is perhaps related to the binding desire of all matter to hold its place as a part of the web of relations.

Water, of which we are mostly constituted, comes from hydrogen, originally, we are told, from the stars. Our earth, a once 'dead' (but now alive with the living) star, our sun, but one of the many living fire stars. Chains of continuity: water, us, the sun, the stars, thermo-nuclear fire, heat, evaporation, water, rain, trees and birds. The sun, a figure in the background of a spatial void, and we – figures beneath the rains that once might have driven us to higher ground – as the moon ever gradually recedes within the chambers of the nautilus shell, we encounter the deserts of our own making.*

* By this I mean that the moon of the ancients, which retained its character and mystery, has receded from us: both literally and metaphorically. Biologists, by observing the daily chamber divisions in nautilus shell fossils, claim that it is possible to determine that at one time the lunar month was only nine days, and therefore it is highly probable that the moon was much closer to the earth. See Daniel B. Botkin, *Discordant Harmonies: A New Ecology for the Twenty First Century* (Oxford: Oxford University Press, 1990), 187.

The second flood has come of our own volition, as a consequence of our own focused cleverness beyond the genius of the bird for flight. It is a flood of noise and images that have no ground, signs that signify nothing but an endless array of vanishings. They signify our bathetic situation, that we must needs continually create to differentiate and hence to orientate; but that creation requires more and more differentiation – there is no God to hold it together, only addiction to progress. The forward orientation of Modernity has, however, run its course, as has the dream of departure. Therefore, I believe we need new metaphors, both visual and performative, that are not based upon the standardizing enterprise of technological light conversion.

The fire from the palette may create ashes or gold, depending upon the orientation of the artist to the subject-matter.

Whether a Luria, a Blake, a Klein, or a Beuys, there is to be found in their diverse work an orientation that lets the light of another, entirely different, qualitative nature in. This light brings alive the metaphor that reorients. The metaphor that reorients is this light. It is nothing, yet it is all.

The metaphor resonates even for a Leonardo – that great old water diviner, who was keenly aware of the mystery of the being/nothingness paradox. Water, as the Zen masters tell us, does not wet water; rather it has its own properties which escape categorization, or representation, and even that of Leonardo's brilliant pen. It forms a world-wide web that retains its material qualities beneath the light speeds of the satellite web above it. There is no 'point' at which it appears and disappears; its oceanic horizon lines expand and contract like a magic balloon in concert with the sun and moon – but it is at war with the earth's only (self-conscious) progenies. We have seen this battle before in the rafts, barques and mirrors of the artists Géricault, Delacroix and Caravaggio. Such encounters with the waters were but visual departure points from which we have long since left.

Should we retrace the desertion or just be content to stand by as Faust's number lands upon the millennium spread-sheet? I certainly don't know – with Descartes I doubt, against Descartes I listen.

I listen for the droplets upon the window frame. They tell me that all is well. If the mirror on to the world is slightly misty, it is just a bit of condensation – it is yet free of prosthetic tubes and light conversion. Though all of this dumb, dirty matter speaks to us of its resistance to acceleration, its desire to be grounded in relation . . . and my palette, another stick, is again wet . . . will it turn to ashes or gold?

With your Tiger Moth joystick and prosthetic drips howling in the clouds over above our earth-bound heads . . . collapsed into a single moment there upon a steel bed in some dark hallway. William Holmes, grandfather, to where would you fly now that you are gone?

My grandmother and I will plant a tree for you.

Landscape of the Psyche: the Dream Theatre of Jenny Kemp

Mark Minchinton with Jenny Kemp

I feel concerned to build alternative structures, completely new structures, new ways of thinking, new ways of perceiving and functioning.

(Jenny Kemp)

Jenny Kemp (b. 1949) is a leading Australian director and writer, who has produced a small number of inno-vative productions of her own (nine plays in seventeen years) and others' playtexts since 1977. She has also been an influential teacher of voice, directing and writing in private workshops and at tertiary training insti-tutions. Her highly structured rehearsal process is based on a refined spatial awareness and visual acuity that owe more to the visual arts than to theatre. Her theatre is built around carefully researched spatial dynamics creating intense fields of energy that rub against her scrupulously constructed vocal and aural texts.

[Kemp's] theatrical collages of visual imagery and soundscapes communicate an impression of sensory realms which flow around each other, inviting the inner responses of the spectators. She sets up a space for the spectators to wander around in with their minds, to roam in, amble through, fantasize about, get lost in, to daydream in.

(Tait *et al.* 1994: 86)

Kemp identifies her father – the eminent painter Roger Kemp, whose abstract work hangs in galleries around the world – as a major influence. As a child Kemp tried to understand the dynamics of his paintings whose power she identifies as coming from their spatial dynamics and energy in relationship to the frame. 'That was a starting-point: having to grapple with that, and having to grapple with the abstraction of the paintings, with metaphysics, and coming to terms with something which is non-representational. That causes one to go inside and look for, or to build, a dialogue inside oneself.'

In its precisely constructed spatial, aural, verbal and visual dynamics her theatre recalls Robert Wilson who has said that 'a small dot in a large room . . . will fill the room simply because of the space around it', and for whom 'a position is a role' (in Cole 1992: 152 and 164).* Kemp's work also recalls that of the American director/writer Maria Irene Fornes (who was a painter before she was a playwright); says Fornes:

* Wilson's words in the citation from Cole come from an interview with Elinor Fuchs (1986) 'The PAJ casebook: Alcestis', *PAJ* 28(10/1): 92–3. The ellipsis in the first citation is Cole's.

If I have a feeling that this actor needs to get up and walk over there, then I don't know if it's right until the actor gets up and does it. . . . [What] guides me on how to block scenes and [in the] composition of scenes . . . has to do with energies that happen between the shapes and persons. Something happens inside the person when the distance between objects and persons changes.

(Fornes in Cole 1992: 47; ellipses and interpolations in original)

Performance Research 3(2), pp.75-87 © Routledge 1998

After early experimental and collaborative work in the late 1970s, Kemp began to map out her concerns with an adaptation of D. M. Thomas's (1981) novel *The White Hotel*, which investigates Freudian psycho-analysis and the slaughter at Babi Yar in 1944. The cataclysmic collision of the inner and outer worlds of (fictional) opera singer Lisa Erdman, whose premonitions of her death at Babi Yar are psychoanalysed by Freud as hysteria, provided ripe material for Kemp's exploration of inner worlds that defy the rationality of the outer world. Kemp went on to write and direct two productions dealing with her own dream material, *Good Night Sweet Dreams* (1986), and *Call of the Wild* (1989) for the Spoleto Festival in Melbourne. With *Call of the Wild* Kemp worked in detail with the paintings of Paul Delvaux, using them as a catalyst for *mise-en-scène*; Delvaux continues to be central to her work. Kemp's next play, *Remember* (1993), which she also directed, departed from autobiographical concerns in examining the events surrounding a woman's rape, subsequent murder of her assailant, and recovery. *Remember* repeated Kemp's concern with the place and power of the internal worlds of memory and dreams, and their interaction with the outer world of 'reality', through complex and closely choreographed repetitions and simultaneous action, interspersed with songs and dance routines by a two-person vaudevillian 'chorus'. Her last work (1996) was *The Black Sequin Dress** commissioned for the Adelaide Festival; it continued her concern with the psychic landscape through repeatedly examining the moment of a woman's entering a nightclub and falling down.

* See the Credit note at the end of this article.

Kemp's focus on the relationship between inner and outer worlds obviously owes much to Jungian analysis and its development by such therapists as Peter O'Connor (1992) and James Hillman (1990). Her concern with inner dialogues, precise use of space, and a blurring of the boundaries between inside and outside, character and character, character and actor have caused many critics to label her work 'Surrealist'. While

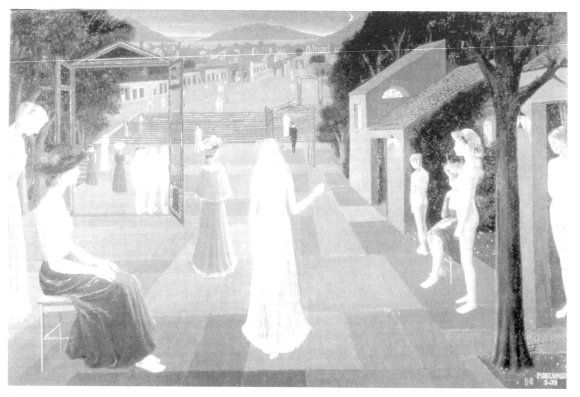

Paul Delvaux, *The Road to Rome*, 1979. Courtesy of Foundation Paul Delvaux

Kemp's interest in the unconscious, her use of fragmented narrative and occasional quotation from other sources to link the apparently banal with the mythic, and her efforts to displace temporal and spatial boundaries seem to invite this label, she herself strongly resists it. Her refusal of the label 'Surrealist' is supported by Alan Read who writes:

> The problem of Surrealism for an ethics of performance . . . is that in the celebration of 'coincidence' and the 'marvellous' was lost the real which was supposed to be superseded by the surreal. Surrealism marked an escape from the everyday not a return to it, a belittling of most people's existence in a process familiar to other avant-gardes predicated on minority status. Though influential within cultural parameters the claims of Surrealism were much more ambitious . . . these claims were not only unfounded but dangerous: 'the real world is accepted since it is transposed instead of being transformed by knowledge'. The Surrealists' revolt against 'the prose of the world' became simply that, a battery of literary techniques.
>
> (Read 1993: 77)*

> * The citation following the ellipsis is from Henri Lefebvre, *Critique of Everyday Life* (London: Verso, 1991), 123.

Kemp's own work is more than just a battery of literary techniques: she attempts to recontextualize what she sees as two essential and connected realms of human experience, the everyday and the inner voices of the psyche. Her aim is not merely to transpose the 'everyday' and 'dream' worlds, but to transform her audience through the knowledge of their unavoidable imbrication. Her political project is quite clear in her interviews:

> Very often, theatre is dealing with overt social concerns. I suppose I feel that the danger and it's why I'm not very satisfied with the theatre that exists is that it doesn't offer something new. It often presents our known structures and offers a critique of them, but in presenting those structures, I often feel they get reinforced.
>
> (Kemp cited in Barrowclough 1995: 26)

This project expresses itself in her sophisticated rehearsal techniques built on an acute recognition of the moment of change, and the part she has to play as an 'observer' in creating that moment.

I have known Jenny Kemp for many years and worked with her as an actor in Call of the Wild *and as a script consultant to* Remember. *The following interview is constructed from conversations in December 1993 and January 1998.*

Mark Minchinton: What was your training background?

Jenny Kemp: Probably the first thing I should mention is my father's influence as a visual artist. Throughout childhood I was confronted with abstract paintings. I spent a lot of time looking at those, trying to find a way of being able to look at them. They largely represent a sense of frameup. I've come to understand it as spatial dynamics and energy in relationship to the frame. That was a starting-point, having to grapple with that, and having to grapple with the abstraction of the paintings, with metaphysics, and coming to terms with something which is non-representational. That causes one to go inside and look for, or to build, a dialogue inside oneself. I had a dialogue with him throughout that time – he largely spoke a language that I didn't quite understand as a child – so I had to try and understand that. I chose not to go into the visual arts because so many people in the family had. It felt like a solitary life and I was more interested in being in relationship to people. I went to the National Institute of Dramatic Arts in Sydney as an actor when I was 17. I only stayed there a year; I felt strongest when I was looking at and critiquing other people's work. I went on being an actor for a number of years, went to England and acted in the fringe, some touring children's theatre companies, and finally an experimental American production, *Liquid*

Theatre, which started me questioning why I was in theatre. I actually gave it away for a number of years and worked on visual art. Then I returned to theatre by training on voice work with Rowena Balos in Australia. That was the beginning of the next phase. I became interested in the voice and realized I was much more interested in the actor from outside than being an actor myself. That was the turn-around: I realized I was quite a good teacher and potentially a good director.

Could we look at your concern with time – both in the works themselves and your rehearsal of them? I'm interested, too, in your use of paintings by a European male of the 1920s and 1930s – Paul Delvaux – to open up, or represent, an Australian female inner landscape in the 1990s. And also talk about internal states . . .

Well, they're not internal states, they're internal actions. My focus at the moment is on internal action: what's happening and able to happen within an internal landscape. Often theatre has been concerned with external action . . . to create the space for a relationship with internal action I've had to address time. To become internally active, society's linear time frame needs to be arrested. We have to depart from cause and effect, beginning, middle and end; to stop travelling in a horizontal direction and open up a vertical time frame. In vertical time we exist in a space where past, present and future coexist; a space where there are states of being to do with memory, dream, reflection, emotion, imagination, simultaneity and psychic phenomena. My interest in these areas is primarily an interest in the creative capacity of the psyche. James Hillman says: 'We gain breadth of soul and wider horizons through vertical descent, through the inwardness of the image.'

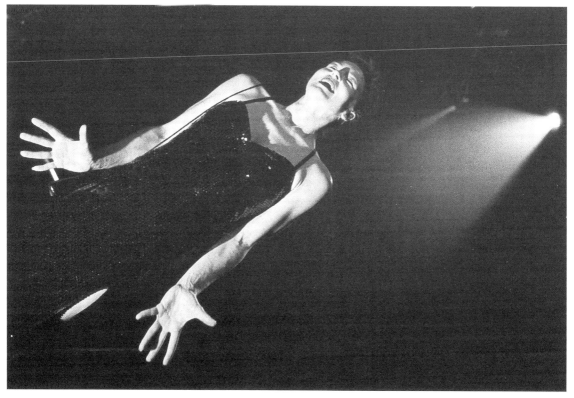

Margaret Mills in *The Black Sequin Dress*, Playbox Theatre Company, Melbourne, 1996. Photo: Jeff Busby

Can I ask whose internal action? You're creating events where the audience is allowed into vertical time, a contemplative, meditative, desire-filled space – and you have to create that same sort of space on stage through rigorous control of the image, the word, and the performers.

Yes, that's right. It's important to remember my background in visual art where the relationship of the viewer to the artwork is very different: the work is stationary, an image. It's always interested me that the still image can cause activity/movement in the viewer, can activate the viewer. What I've found problematic, often, is that when theatre is very active the audience becomes passive, is *acted upon*. I want theatre that allows the audience to be much more active. I'm pulling away from work being an 'active' thing and introducing elements that make the audience stop moving forward. The audience's impulse is to keep moving forward, to look for the action and what happens next, but in *The Black Sequin Dress*, for instance, there was little dramatic action, the audience's forward movement was arrested and they were made to continually look at one moment: the only way they could move was 'vertically'.

Would any moment do for that? It's a very specific moment in *Black Sequin Dress* – a woman falls down in a nightclub. How do you choose the moment?

Well, it's partly personal, isn't it? That moment came from reading about someone lying on a kitchen floor, and I had a memory from when I was about 12 of my mother lying on a kitchen floor and I thought she was dead. So falling had particular impact for me, and the connection with the descent myth of Persephone seemed strong. And there's a fantastic disjunction between the sophisticated woman and the act of falling like a child. And the idea of the fallen woman – I mean there's all that. It's quite a powerful gestalt even though, or because, to fall over is an ordinary event. However, theoretically it seems to me that *any* action could have extraordinary resonance. In terms of vertical time or the Aboriginal concept of the eternal now, where the past continues to exist in the present, then any moment is absolutely full. Part of the dilemma of the fast-forward, fast-moving, fast-food consuming society is that any particular moment is empty, there's a grasping for the next moment because this one's dispensed with and eaten up and chewed and spat out. You can stop in any moment, anywhere, and it will be full, and the 'history' of that moment will be alive.

There's a tension, isn't there, between the desire to create a contemplative moment and the kind of 'lens' that allows that to happen: the lens you use is highly wrought and constructed.

Well, to pinpoint a moment requires a lot of control. To clarify: I started off saying I was interested in internal action, but I'm not interested in that in isolation – it's its relationship with external action. I'm looking at how what's happening internally is in disjunction with external 'reality'. To look at that relationship requires control: finding how they're connected at any moment is not a generalized thing, it's not interesting if it's generalized – I'm interested in the particular.

Your rehearsal work is very finely detailed; maybe you could talk about how you arrive at that detail. The Delvaux paintings are particularly interesting because they're very theatrical in themselves – someone else might simply animate them, but you don't do that.

Recognizing the links between memory, physicality and emotion – there's often a tilt of the head or some tension through the body that triggers it – with the paintings, the text and the theatre space, I'm looking for a particular relationship where it synthesizes with my own internal landscape. With the paintings it's to do with the spatial dynamics which have a particular emotional field/feel to them. The paintings seem to be only partially to do with the everyday world, they evoke another world, another landscape, an inner landscape. It's something to do with how a spatial dynamic causes an emotional dynamic: when I work with the actor, when she or he is in a particular position with a particular tension, that causes a gestalt to open up, or to drop through on the vertical level. I'm looking for the stage moment to have a multiplicity of meanings. When James Hillman analogizes the dream image and asks, 'What is it like?', he says keep working with the image so that it has many possibilities, many meanings. I'm looking for the moment when many resonances are possible. That's where it gets exciting, and that's a lot to do with how I read the stage action visually.

Paintings are two-dimensional objects which you have the illusion of looking into; likewise, your theatre is a theatre you look into not across. It's hard to imagine it in the round. We did *Call of the Wild* on a slight thrust stage on tour in Sydney and that was quite difficult. Once you shift from looking from one side of a spatial relationship to another side, the relationships and the emotional field all change.

If I'm working with an image what's important is the relationship of the figure to the architecture, and the figure to the space, and if we pull it out into the round it's another ball game; it's not something you can contemplate. The spectator is like the dreamer watching their dream, and I like that relationship – that someone's dreaming it. What does a dream look like? We know it isn't linear, the images are happening simultaneously; when we tell a dream we organize it linearly.

Dream space is like the Tardis in *Doctor Who* – the space is bigger inside than outside.

When you look at something on stage, you look at it and you're out here, and then you zoom in. Videoing a stage show flattens it out, and makes you realize when you're watching a show your eye is continually zooming in. You're watching the whole thing but latching on to and entering a moment. Coming back to Delvaux – someone looking at the paintings with a feminist critique might be critical of them, but I see the women as quite empowered within them: because of the number of women in the frame, and because they're larger and more present than the men. The men are small, less luminous, and quite ugly, they're imploding; the women are empowered because they're involved in their own meditation. Maybe one of the major links as a person living by the sea in Melbourne is that there are trams in the paintings! And the sea! What's fascinating in the paintings are the disjunctions between the banal and the everyday (which don't look banal in his paintings – trams look like extraordinary presences!). The time gap between his painting and me now is irrelevant, because what I'm relating to is that he's shifted himself outside time. If I use the paintings years later in Australia it doesn't matter, I never felt a difference. I don't know what's particularly European about him or what's particularly Australian about me. I don't know the answer to that, because I feel like I've never quite known the answer to that. Sometimes I've tried to answer the question for myself and felt that I'm perhaps provoked by the lack of external action in this country so you find something internal! Or perhaps it's the 'emptiness' of the desert! [*Laughs.*] Riding the tram out through the suburbs of Brussels it didn't feel that different – there were supermarkets and people doing their shopping, it felt pretty much the same as here!

I'd like to come back to what drives your decision-making process conceptually.

Practically, writing the text is separate from the writing of the scenic action. That's more like drawing a storyboard. Personally, I've needed to come to terms with internal chaos and to live with it, to live alongside it, not ditch it, but to dialogue with it; and to recognize the disjunctive existence we have with what is at the surface a highly organized, constructed society with this massive chaotic element inside. I want to sort out that relationship and to get it functioning creatively, to make accessible and functional those inner resources which are heavily repressed socially. Possibly, this is particularly important to me because of dealing with mental illness in my near family. The writing tends to be triggered by . . . I just like writing . . . I like the process of writing . . . I like the process of the pen on the page. I used to draw – writing's a bit like drawing. What I'm doing in the moment of writing is seeing what my unconscious has to say. Just trying to open up and not control what comes out because I feel over-dominated by the conscious mind, so it's a chance to see what's inside. Writing's a chance to see what's happening now, so I can start having a relationship with it. Being conscious about it and naming it is an important part of the maturation process. I write best when I give a writing workshop and we work every day for a week from 10 a.m. to 3 p.m.: I approach the workshop saying I'm not going to write because I don't want to write from that conscious place – I might do that later once the big offer is out – then I usually do the writing exercise anyway! The best thing is to be surprised by what comes out, and not to recognize it after. Then there's a huge task after to see the pattern the writing presents, to be conscious of what it is and identify what it's about; and then write further consciously.

That's interesting, because I've meant to ask you about presentation, representation, and recognition, and I was wondering about recognition?

. . . the process of recognition?

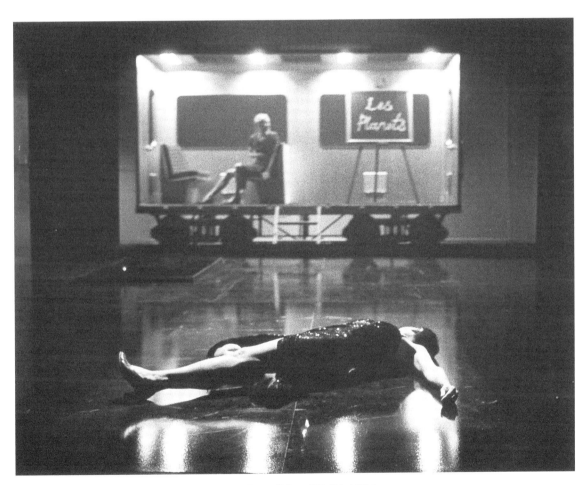

Natasha Herbert and Helen Herbertson in *The Black Sequin Dress*, Playbox Theatre Company, Melbourne, 1996. Photo: Jeff Busby

Yes, because theatre audiences are so tuned to plotlines, characters, stories, and so on, you challenge their recognition. Sometimes they may not recognize what sort of event you're dealing with. And you need to recognize what the writing event is.

It's difficult. In the new work I'm working on, *Still Angela*, I'm working on about eight different streams. A couple of those will end up being irrelevant – I've got to be careful in identifying the relevant ones. I've got to ask what is the key image or key action here, and then be able to tell you it in one sentence, like I can now with *The Black Sequin Dress*: 'a woman comes into a nightclub and falls over'. I have to contextualize it in a way that's accessible and recognizable. The storyboard is another process that comes afterward when the action is identified. Because I'm interested in the relation-ship between the everyday, the here and now, and the other, I've got to acknowledge the everyday includes narrative structure, social time frame, and so on – I've got to work with them. It could be that an image from a painting helps me to identify the action. I'm looking for an action and a context from which text can be spoken . . . and if the characters are often speaking from the unconscious where do they speak it from? Are they at a kitchen table? Or are they eating dinner? Walking down a road? Where and how are they, and what are they doing? And there's something about those paintings that reminds me of what's possible. That makes the unconscious a tangible embodied place.

That's interesting that you've asked where and how, you've not asked who they are.

Who the people are?

Yes, is that a question for you?

Yes, it is. But the paintings help me to address location; and it always feels that in some way location is a landscape of the psyche, so it's an internal landscape but it's got to have a groundedness about it. It's got to have both aspects but if it gets too grounded it gets too tight, and if it gets too far from that no one knows where we are, it floats off. If you look at those paintings it often looks like all the women are the same woman, and all the men the same man and – coming back to the idea that the audience is the dreamer – then everyone in the dream is at any moment an aspect of themselves. For me they're always the same person; all the women are the same woman. In *The Black Sequin Dress* they were all different ages but they could have been the same woman at different times in her life. But it wasn't that explicit. When I was directing, I felt there was a certain sort of sexual energy that I wanted on stage, to focus on, and part of casting was trying to pinpoint that energy. And the men feel to me like they're part of a psyche too – as you know!

This process – writing, storyboarding, and then directing – is from your perspective seamless: has anyone else done your plays, and do you think they could be done by someone else?

No one else has produced them. It feels like I'm completing the writing by directing it. But all the collaborations I've had – such as with (composer) Elizabeth Drake, (choreogra-pher) Helen Herbertson, (designer) Jacqui Everitt – have allowed another dynamic to enter. It feels important that I don't have too much control.

I've wanted to ask about performers – given your love of, need for, precise physical detail and control in your performers, would dancers be better for your work?

It's interesting, that idea of control. I suspect all the storyboarding, and the amount of control I've had to have in rehearsal, has been partly economically driven. On a long rehearsal period we have six weeks. I had to fight for my six weeks on *Black Sequin Dress* (this is for a major festival production), they were going to give me four or five. I work solidly on the storyboards in order to have an offer to make to the actors; the world that the text sits within is not explicit from the text itself – you don't read it and think, ah yes, this is a naturalistic thriller, or whatever – you don't know what it is. I have to say, OK this is the world that it is, this is a landscape where time doesn't exist, and this is the feel of it, look at these pictures, here's an example of what could happen here. I have to make a strong and particular offer in order to bring them all into the same world. I'd be very happy to use a less explicit starting-point if we had time. I'd say, here are the elements, have a look at this, let's see what you offer up. To a certain extent that does happen in rehearsal and we deviate from the storyboard; the storyboard doesn't always work, it makes things a bit tight, too controlled. I would love to get away from that, but what can I do? When I worked in the dance world I felt released because we were able to work for twelve weeks on image. I felt this is right, this is how long it takes. Dancers know that, they're writing their texts in their bodies. Now for some reason theatre has got so that it's expected that rehearsal is about the text, it's not about the movement very often; it's changing, but many actors are still just thinking about the text. Dancers' capacity for the particular in relation to their bodies and the image is endless, and really good actors will work like that.

But what about that thing you see in many dancers where they might be physically particular, but they don't have a world going?

Yes, nice little pieces but there's nothing going on.

Nothing going on between the people in the space.

Or between the people and the space, or the place. Yes, how do you get to the epic without narrative?

By 'epic' you mean?

The closest I've got to it is calling something an experiential narrative. You engage someone on a journey through their psyche, that they can't walk away from – they'd be halfway through a gestalt. Instead of the death of the soldier or the princess it's the death of your old self!

If people thought that was going to happen no one would go!

Yes, well it is a bit tricky! I saw Teshigawara at the London International Festival of Theatre and his piece had a sense of travelling through landscape after landscape after landscape; a major journey was being taken where, in narrative terms, we ended up in the inner sanctum and coming out the other end, back to the everyday, to the natural world. Maybe dance is the place you can do narrative best, because it's so abstract it's in disjunction with it.

Jude Walton once pointed out that 'sexy' dance is often not sexual so much as a demonstration of sexuality; she asked how do you keep the desire between dancers real, what would that type of dance be? And we thought it would require of the dancers a commitment that they're not used to giving, because so much of dance calls for a fetishizing of . . .

. . . form.

Yes, now it seems to me you're asking of your actors that they . . .

. . . fetishize the form. [*Laughs.*]

And that they bring the possibility of their everyday selves being there.

Yes, they're not playing characters.

They're just . . .

. . . present.
When I work with actors, what's most important is that
they really relax. Even if we haven't got lots of time it's
very important in the early rehearsal to remove the time
pressure altogether, to give the illusion of incredible
space and time. When you do that the first part's quite
slow, but then the actors can work quickly because
they're coming from a creative state. I hope that the
formality of my structures enables actors to feel secure
enough to be utterly vulnerable within them. If they
know they're going to walk, they know they're going to
walk along that line with their hips at this angle and
their shoulders at that angle. And we know what that's
about, we've found exactly what tensions the body holds
to locate the emotional state that is right for the text.
What's happening physically is tangible, that's where
you relate. When the actor hits the emotional, balanced
state where she or he's whole, then I'll try to describe
her precisely; and I'll probably give her some text
instantly, because that's where the language needs to
come from. It's a state of being. When we come to
repeat it I'll ask what she was working on. Often it's

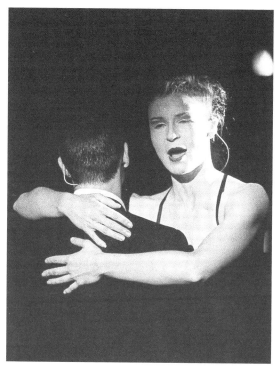

Margaret Mills and Greg Stone in *The Black Sequin Dress*, Playbox Theatre Company,
Melbourne, 1996. Photo: Jeff Busby

something I set up, for example, the state of pain. We can work on an active verb (remembering, fantasizing, and
so on) or a state of being (pain, anger, or whatever). We'll go through it again, and she ends up sitting on the
seat, that's where she's landed herself, so we'll keep that in. The next time she sits I might notice, say, that she
hasn't got her hands on her knees, she's sitting back not forward, she's looking straight ahead not down, her
hands are beside her body, and the state isn't there. I'll say put your hands on your knees, lean forward, and look
down. She does that and it unlocks the state again. Sometimes we have to go back to the exact physical state.
When the state is solidly landed she might be able to deviate physically a little bit but it's fragile at the start.
Often people resist relocating something unfamiliar, they have to go to exactly the same position and relax, then
it'll unlock. We find a physical manifestation of an emotional/mental state that is registered perceptively in a
physical position. Time and time again the actor will go back and her body won't necessarily remember, and I'll
have to remind her of the exact shape. Rationally she'll be telling herself that she's going to do something else
now, be a bit 'creative', that there's no point doing the same thing again, and so on.

**So your job as the director is to encourage the actors to allow themselves to go to the state, and to
remember the physical detail?**

To reassure. Instead of saying, 'I need you to find an emotional state
where you'll be quite fragile' – an actor can't find that – it's much easier to say, 'We were working on "reflect-
ing"; sit on that chair, lift your head a bit, it's there somewhere, just feel it.' It should be simple. With detailed
physical instructions actors at best have a sense of security, at worst they feel trapped. There's a particular kind
of actor who can handle that: an actor who is able to work vertically. If you put parameters around them, restrictions on them, they'll go down, they'll go in; whereas if you put restrictions on other actors they feel paralysed,

straitjacketed, because they're not prepared to go into the depth, not prepared to open up into the chaos. A lot of times the most exciting emotional state has a slight element of the unknown in it, it's right on an edge.

But you're not dealing with purely emotional states, are you?

No, it might be the state of reflection, remembering, or fantasizing. But we need to locate how the *particular* performer locates that state. These aren't necessarily familiar states that actors are used to working with. It's to do with timing and rhythm, because I work a lot with impulse; they're the key things in relation to the text. When the actor has located the state of remembering, for instance, it's got a particular rhythm for her. I can't tell her what her rhythm is because my rhythm will be different; it's important that we find her rhythm because that will be interesting. It's a lot to do with actors finding a relationship to their own timing. I impose a whole lot of things but I don't impose that.

How do you avoid manufacturing and controlling the action totally?

I've had to confront that a lot because of working with the Delvaux paintings. I look at the paintings and there's a particular spatial dynamic, which includes a figure who is in a

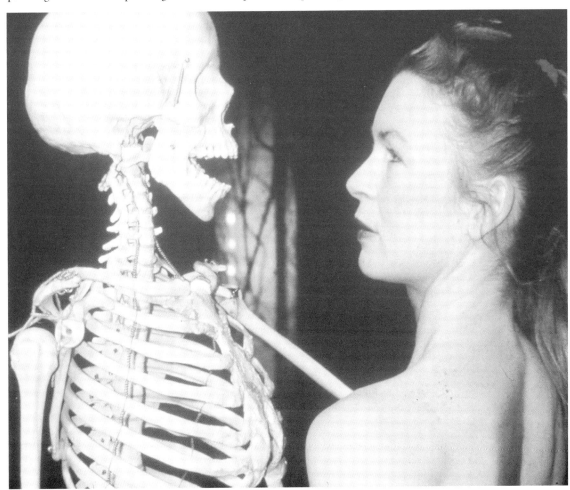

Credit: Margaret Mills in *Call of the Wild* (1989) dir. Jenny Kemp
Photo: Jeff Busby

particular dynamic with another figure in relation to the architecture. I believe in giving the actor a lot of freedom, but I've had to work out another way where I can say, 'I want you in this position'. I have to work with great care so the actor also has freedom to explore outside that position. What I might do is say, 'This is the position I want you to end up in, but this is the journey we can take to end up there; that might enable you to be open, once you get that position.' I can't just say, 'Sit there and be like that!', bang, bang, bang. I can say what we're going for and show them the painting, but then we have to undertake the work to give the actor the internal freedom to find that position. Once they've got the position, they then need an equal amount of freedom to feel back through the body into themselves from that position, to be receptive and responsive to the spatial dynamic I'm giving them. When you're working around the other way you give them freedom and they find the position that arrives out of that. If I give them the position, I still have to give them the freedom to go back the other way. Or I give them a journey to arrive at a particular point. It's tricky, and it's something I've had to really confront. I work from both angles, not always from givens. Mostly the story-boards from the paintings are starting-points only.

What's the difference between directing your own work and directing someone else's work?

With text that's given to me I need to work very solidly conceptually and visually, to find a world to give the actors parameters within which to land. In some ways that's not hugely different from my own work where I do have a shift-over point from writing into the storyboard phase which is an act of creation comparable to that of creating the text. Sometimes with a text that's given to me I draw a storyboard and work off paintings. It mightn't be quite as pinned down as some of my story-boards for my own work, but even the storyboards for my own work are only starting-points. The actors are more dependent on me in my work, they don't know what the world is going to be, it's not as apparent from the text where I'm going. Often with someone else's script, it's a more recognizable world to the actors in some way because it's derived more directly from a social context, so they know where they are: they're in a room with furniture, or in a kitchen, having a conversation with a person in a particular sort of way. But what about when you're communicating a thought-state or a dream-state? That's another task, I try to be specific about how the actual world on stage will manifest. The actors need that to be quite specifically pinned down or they're going to be really lost . . . of course, as a director these days scripts are becoming much more challenging in this respect.

Do you feel lonely in the Australian theatre scene? We're in a country with a population probably equal to Greater London's or New York's, there's not a lot of work of the kind you're talking about.

I think I'd feel lonely anywhere. The work's dialoguing with, is about, being alone. There's a sprinkling of other works in the world. Hotel Pro Forma's *Operation Orfeo* [see *Performance Research* 1(3) (1996)] was very reinforcing for me because Kirsten Dehlholm was working with visual elements in a way that I found interesting. I felt slightly less lonely watching that, but is anyone else working like that in her country? Twenty years ago I spent four years in London and I certainly didn't find anything there that made me feel less lonely. But when I came back my loneliness, or aloneness, or the sense of loneliness one can feel in this country, was a catalyst in my work.

ACKNOWLEDGEMENTS
Credits for *The Black Sequin Dress*

Writer and Director:	Jenny Kemp	Music:	Elizabeth Drake
Designer:	Jacqui Everitt	Lighting:	Ben Cobham

Cast: Natasha Herbert/Helen Herbertson/Margaret Mills/Ian Scott/Mary Sitarenos/Greg Stone
My thanks to Tania Angelini at Playbox Theatre, Jeff Busby and David Williams for their assistance with this article. Especial thanks to Jenny Kemp for making the time to be interviewed.

REFERENCES

Barrowclough, N. (1995) 'Theatre of dreams', *The Good Weekend: The Age Magazine* (supplement to the Melbourne Age) (16 September): 22–7.

Cole, S. L. (1992) *Directors in Rehearsal: a Hidden World*, New York and London: Routledge.

Hillman, J. (1990) *The Essential James Hillman: A Blue Fire*, London: Routledge.

Kemp, J. (1989) '*Call of the Wild*', in Karen Pearlman and Richard James Allen (eds) *Performing the Unnamable: an Anthology of Australian Texts in Performance*, Sydney: Currency Press and Real Time, forthcoming (1998).

Kemp, J. (1993) '*Remember*', in Peta Tait and Elizabeth Schafer (eds) *Australian Women's Drama: Texts and Feminisms*, Sydney: Currency Press, 1997.

Kemp, J. (1996) *The Black Sequin Dress*, Sydney: Currency Press and Playbox Theatre.

O'Connor, P. (1992[1986]) *Dreams and the Search for Meaning*, Port Melbourne: Mandarin.

Read, A. (1993) *Theatre and Everyday Life: An Ethics of Performance*, London and New York: Routledge.

Tait, Peta *et al.* (1994) *Converging Realities: Feminism in Australian Theatre*, Sydney: Currency Press in conjunction with Artmoves.

Thomas, D. M. (1981) *The White Hotel: a Novel*, London: Gollancz.

Performing the unnameable
An Anthology of Australian Performance Texts
Edited by Richard James Allen and Karen Pearlman

A co-publication with RealTime, this is the first collection of performance texts created by Australian performers, performance companies and writers. *Performing the Unnameable* pays tribute to the largely undocumented work of a generation of artists working across the boundaries of theatre, performance, performance art and new media. Spanning a twenty-year period, and including over 20 outstanding texts, the collection includes work by The Sydney Front, Open City, Jenny Kemp, Lyndal Jones, Sidetrack Performance Group, Richard Murphet, Margaret Cameron, Josephine Wilson, Legs on the Wall, Entr'Acte and many others.

As well as production notes and photographs, there will also be an introduction from each of the artists/writers documenting their observations on the works in performance. The texts are revealing about the contribution of words to performance, their relationship with design, choreography, music, sound, new media and other artforms.

This unique anthology is a much needed resource for practitioners, teachers, students and audiences of Australian performance.

About the Editors. Richard James Allen & Karen Pearlman have been working in the areas of performance, writing and filmmaking since the early 1980s. Their works have been performed, published and screened widely on three continents. Their broad-ranging experience and interests in both live and print media inspired them to undertake the documentation of a generation of texts in performance which might otherwise disappear.

Performing the Unnameable will be published in September by Currency Press, the Australian Performing Arts Publisher. isbn: 0 86818 420 4; rrp $35 (approx); 224 pages (approx); format: 275 x 215 mm; illustrations in b/w.
For further information please contact Deborah Franco at Currency Press.
Tel: 61 (0) 2 9319 5877 Fax: 61 (0) 2 9319 3649
e-mail: currency@magna.com.au
www.currency.com.au

Abstraction has many Faces: the Ballet/Modern Wars of Lincoln Kirstein and John Martin

Mark Franko

Is a Rockette a little rock? Or, is it a little rocket? Is it *little*? . . . Later: Someone has just told me that a Rockette is a little Rockefeller.

(Waring 1967)

In the last few years, as if in a strange time-warp, I have witnessed reconstructions of dance works from the 1930s receive enthusiastic responses from contemporary audiences.* Anyone wishing to know about the full repertory soon discovers, however, that only a few dances actually survive. Scattered mentions in reviews and an occasional photograph are all that remain of the majority of politically radical modern dances of the 1930s. Despite the recent rediscovery of left-wing critic Edna Ocko and her lucid discussions of radical performance, there is no body of writing that deals exhaustively with the dances.† Living memories are also fading and many of the oral histories recorded between the 1960s and the 1980s tend to underplay the political significance of 1930s dance, a significance that it had not yet

* See, in particular, Eve Gentry's *Tenant of the Streets* in the 1993 New Dance Group Retrospective Concert (available on video from the American Dance Guild, New York City), the reconstruction of Martha Graham's *Panorama* by the Martha Graham Dance Company, and Jane Dudley's concert at the Place, London, *Dated* (available on video from Singh Productions, London).

† See Ocko 1994; and Edna Ocko, 'From a Conversation with Edna Ocko' and 'The Revolutionary Dance Movement', in Franko (1995: 33–7, 124–7).

become fashionable to address head on. This state of affairs leads the persistent researcher to ask what position the two major dance writers of the early twentieth century – Lincoln Kirstein and John Martin – took on radical dance, or, at least, how radical dance was positioned in their work.

This essay does just that, and addresses in the process the relation of ideology to mainstream dance criticism and theory in the 1930s. It questions the famous tension between ballet and modern that Kirstein and Martin enacted in the critical arena and bequeathed to posterity as representative of authentic ideological strife. Did the ballet/modern wars not rather serve to depoliticize dance in print, making conflict an internalized and aestheticized affair? This essay proposes that the real scene of ideological strife took place between modern dancers and chorus girls for whom ballet dancers in America of the 1930s were the surrogates.‡ How this was so can become clear from a close reading of Kirstein's project for the construction of an American ballet in the radical decade.

‡ For a discussion of high and low in American performance, see Levine 1988.

I

While radical modern dance tried to address the masses during the 1930s, classical ballet in America also sought a broad popular base. Self-ordained apologist and well-endowed patron of the new American ballet Lincoln Kirstein competed with a then influential left culture for the idea of a 'mass audience'.* Refusing to imagine his desired spectators as snobbish or elite, Kirstein hypothesized that the average American consumer of popular culture could become a balletomane. If only ballet could be made to reflect the clichéd content of movies and newspapers, everyday folk would want to see it. The Russian ballet then dominated American touring circuits, and their flamboyant style was associated with ballet art in the American mind. Kirstein denounced the Russian ballet hegemony vigorously as 'the Great Conspiracy' that robbed his plan for an American ballet of its native audience. In polemicizing home-grown ballet versus foreign imports, Kirstein focused on the necessity to eradicate a certain kind of ballet, viewed by a certain kind of public, and performed by certain kinds of dancers. His overarching argument was to retain the integrity of 'international theatrical dancing' – the 400-year-old classical pedagogy of dance technique. The ballet idea for Kirstein was transhistorical and 'absolute'. He not only asserted that ballet was a timeless although still evolving training method for theatrical movement, but also projected that ballet was capable of absorbing and abstracting elements foreign to its own basic sources such as movements from non-European cultures as well as themes or musics not associated with ballet history. Retaining its integrity, ballet assimilated elements foreign to its own European balletic logic. Nevertheless, Kirstein was not entirely traditional in that he looked to the Diaghilev era for inspiration, and particularly to the modernist choreography of Vaslav Nijinsky.

Although Kirstein salvaged American ballet's

* Kirstein published two articles in the left-wing magazine *New Theatre* in which he blandly defended the contemporary relevance to the masses of classical ballet technique (Kirstein 1934 and 1935).

social relevance, its technical adaptability, and its modernism, he was tied above all to a classical *form*, and was committed to argue that the technical basis of that form could be adapted to fit unusual content. Thus the importance in Kirstein's mind of 'popular vaudeville, revue-dance, and popular jazz or swing music' for the development of American ballet (Kirstein 1937: 246†). These styles could be sufficiently abstracted by the classical form to fashion an aesthetically acceptable if ersatz popular culture. Since the subject-matter of American ballet was to be drawn from popular culture, the forms of elegance and personality associated with dance classicism would have to be modified. Kirstein called this modification 'grafting'.

† Further references to this pamphlet will be given by bracketed page numbers in the text.

The presumed affinity of classical ballet for American popular performance culture is not a purely conjectural construct on Kirstein's part. Ballet in America has a history connecting it with popular culture. In the Ziegfeld film *Glorifying the American Girl* (1929), chorus girl Gloria Hughes (Mary Eaton) auditions for the Follies using the outdated shuffling numbers she learned from her ageing Vaudeville partner. Fearing rejection, she pleads with the rehearsal director to show what she alone can 'really do'. Given another chance, she performs an impromptu ballet variation in pointe shoes which succeeds in landing her a starring role in the Follies. As I interpret this segment, classical ballet was a way of moving that the chorus girl never studied, but rather discovered as a native resource in herself. Classical ballet, in more general terms, belonged to the chorus girl's mythical cultural capital. The permeability between ballet and show dance testified to by this myth lent credibility to Kirstein's project for an indigenous American ballet. Yet, in his writing, he presents it as an idea without historical precedent.

One can point to further precedents for this cultural affinity. The balletic choreographic tradition of the Follies was linked to popular ballets of the late nineteenth century such as *The Black*

Crook (1866) just as 'nineteenth-century ballet spectacles had engendered the image of the American chorus girl' (Hardy 1980: 119).* The chorus girl was a figure of popular American culture linked

* 'From the term "ballet girl",' writes Hardy, 'came the slightly disreputable aura that attached itself to the chorus girl as her identity emerged' (1980: 102).

to the call girl, but also to the 'ballet girl'. Behind the American ballet dancer stood Lydia Thompson's British Blonds, the Gibson Girls, the Tiller Girls – all of whom, like Anna Pavlova, toured the States – not to mention the Ziegfeld Follies, which began in New York in 1907. There is also a high art connection of the Follies, Michael Fokine – one of Diaghilev's Ballets Russes choreographers who settled in America in 1919. Fokine's first commission in the new world was to

choreograph the musical *Aprodite*. In 1922, Fokine contributed two numbers to the Ziegfeld Follies (see Horwitz 1985: 57–72). Pointe shoes and feathers are trappings of *The Dying Swan*, his legendary 1905 solo for Anna Pavlova, as well as of the Follies soft-focus girlie spectacle of the early 1930s (Figure 1). During the 1930s, the ultimate Kirstein protégé George Balanchine devised choreography in New York for the Ziegfeld Follies of 1936 and in Hollywood for the film *Goldwyn Follies* (1938), as well as for Broadway musicals. Kirstein does not emphasize these facts, looking instead on the work of European dance modernists in commercial American theater as a mild dilution of their authentic values. What he never calls into question, however, is the cultural continuity of practices underpinning this conjuncture. More is at issue

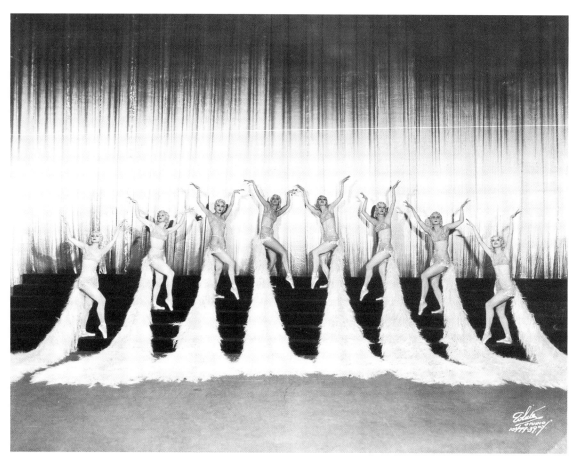

Figure 1: A 1931 Ziegfeld Follies production number in which pointe shoes, the hallmarks of classical ballet, are combined with feather boas, the hallmarks of burlesque. Courtesy of the Billy Rose Theater Collection, New York Public Library for the Performing Arts at Lincoln Center, Astor, Lenox and Tilden Foundations

here than the locations of display. These, it seems, were fairly loose; they permitted Martha Graham and Harald Kreutzberg to present modern dance at the gala opening of Radio City Music Hall in 1932. The historical interconnection of classical ballet and commercial theater dance, however, was something entirely different: it testifies to a collusion not only of occasions and locations but also of practices – both technical and thematic – with a settled historical basis in American performance. Classical ballet had existed in American musical theater since the late nineteenth century. The first permanent American ballet company was the Radio City Music Hall Company established in 1932 as an adjunct to the Rockettes (Francisco 1979: 84). Ballet modernism in the European tradition of Kazian Goleizovsky, Vaslav Nijinsky and Bronislava Nijinska was a latecomer to American theaters. Balanchine's first independent concert presentation, at which *Serenade* premiered, was in 1935.* In his attempt to invent American ballet in the 1930s, Kirstein overlooked the fact that it had already been invented. His mission was actually to institutionalize it.

The Goldwyn Follies provides a miniature allegory of what Kirstein was after. A European film producer (Adolphe Menjou) overhears a typical American girl (Helen Jepson) accuse his work of artificiality. Realizing that she is a natural taste arbiter, he hires her to advise him on what the American public really wants. In one episode, they sit in a darkened theater/sound-stage watching the filming of Balanchine's choreography for *Romeo and Juliet*. The American girl complains that Romeo and Juliet should be married and live happily ever after. Menjou immediately requests the proper changes. In the choreography itself, the Capulets and the Montagues are all women, but are represented by different dance styles: ballet and show dance. Each group performs a short sequence of choreography and is then supplanted by the other. While this stylistic difference seems to be

* *Serenade* was 'the first work Balanchine choreographed for American dancers'. See *Choreography by George Balanchine. A Catalogue of Works* (1983: 117).

motivated by a conflict between the two families, it also works visually as a counterpoint between the classical and the modern, the old world of Europe and the new world of America. The curtain opens on what looks like a tenement: laundry hangs from clothes-lines extended from building to building over the stage. But when the laundry is brusquely drawn in, a small Italian village square is evoked. Similarly, the dancers are dressed in modern attire until the love duet when the two soloists appear in pseudo-Renaissance garb. The rewritten ending shows show dancers and ballet dancers together, bumping, grinding and pirouetting in modern dress as the laundry lines return. What this choreographic sequence demonstrates is not only the necessity of updating classical ballet to commercial show dance standards, but also the ease and facility with which this can be accomplished. The American public wants them, after all, to live happily ever after.

The connection between commercial theater and classical ballet in American culture remains, none the less, implicit in Kirstein's argument; it was the unspoken foundation for his recourse to American popular culture in the creation of new ballets. In his view classical American dancing needed to display American character, which it could cultivate, in Kirstein's words, after the model of 'American character dancing' as represented by 'vaudeville or musical-comedy' as well as by ballroom dancing.[†] These dancing images were widely disseminated in Hollywood films where Kirstein found another element of national character susceptible to assimilation by ballet: the dancer's personality, or personal style. 'Our style springs from the personal atmosphere of recognizable American types as exemplified by the behavior of movie stars like Ginger Rogers, Carole Lombard, or the late Jean Harlow' [201] (Figure 2).

[†] ibid.: 257. He neglected to note that European classical dancing developed from the roots of character dance. Study of the Renaissance dancing manuals he so often referred to could have revealed to him that classical dance vocabulary was itself adapted from popular vernaculars, the original *materia choreographica* he so often touted. What Kirstein proposed, however, was to append the already historically developed classical technique to contemporary entertainment and thus to display further adapatations of which classical technique was capable.

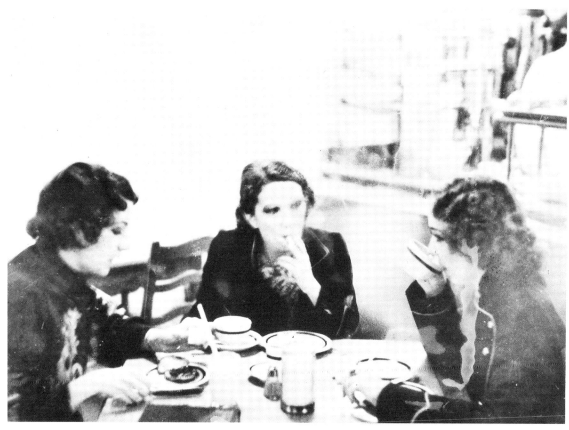

Figure 2: The Rockettes as pajama'd workers in 1936. The photo legend reads: 'Luncheon: the girls eat their meals in the theatre cafeteria – in pajamas if they wish. Here are Betty Sasscier, Ruth Sproule, and Dorothea Frank over their coffee cups.' Courtesy of the Dance Collection, New York Public Library for the Performing Arts at Lincoln Center, Astor, Lenox and Tilden Foundations

More precisely, Kirstein imagined these celebrities as able to 'establish a direct connection, approaching personal intimacy, or its cinematic equivalent, with their audiences'. The example that came first to his mind in 'Blast at ballet' was that of Follies performer Helen Morgan, 'perched on her piano' [201].

Initially the exorcism of foreign influence from national ballet venues was more urgent to Kirstein's project than his rivalry with another home-grown theatrical movement: modern dance. But despite the time and energy he spent attacking European ballet imports, no one did more than Kirstein to popularize the idea of an ideological schism between classical ballet and modern dance. Given the situation just outlined, he did this for reasons as much of political expediency as of aesthetic investment. 'Modern dance', he wrote, 'was a radical

revolt from it [classical theatrical dancing], so violent at its outset that the base was rootless' [254]. For Kirstein, this meant that modern dance disqualified itself as legitimate theater. To deny theatrical legitimacy to modern dance masked the historical continuity between ballet and American popular culture, one in which ballet was subservient to the popular, rather than the other way around. It masked, in other terms, the low culture status of American classical ballet. Kirstein diverted attention from the 'commercial' status of dance forms to issues of their legitimacy, arguing on this basis modern dance's absence of theatricality. Without theatricality, no legitimacy. Although frequently applied to Martha Graham, this flawed argument was the setpiece of his public debate with John Martin, first dance critic of the *New York Times*. Martin's key term in this context was not, however, 'theater', as Kirstein hastily insisted, but rather 'spectacle'. Martin attributed the qualities of spectacle to ballet and the qualities of ritual to modern dance [257].* The spectacle implies personal attendance at impersonal, visual, 'historical' events that represent the decline of ritual and festival *communitas* in human experience. Although Martin did not fully develop the ramifications of his critique of spectacle on behalf of modern dance in either anthropological or political economy terms, such a critique was implicit in his critical vantage point.†

* For further analysis of Martin's position, see Franko 1996. For an account of Martin's institutional identity as dance critic, see Conner 1997.

† For a detailed discussion of this view see MacAloon 1984. On *communitas*, see Turner 1995.

II

Unlike Kirstein, who had the independent means to be a patron of ballet, Martin was a professional dance critic, the first on the staff of the *New York Times*. From his watchtower – his institutional position as critic of a great metropolitan newspaper – Martin willingly (perhaps haphazardly) submitted himself to a series of personal experiments. He attends modern dance concerts, allowing the images he sees there to assail his mind and senses, developing in tandem with his visual and visceral perceptions a quasi-theoretical evaluation of what is happening with respect to what *might* happen, what *could* happen, perhaps even what *should* happen. For all that, he is also a witness reporting that something *did* happen, documenting the historical density of sounds and bodies in motion together with his own presence at these historical events.

Martin's lack of enthusiasm for the 'spectacular' aspects of classical ballet and his constant emphasis on the emotion modern dance can transmit cause his writing to appear aligned with the left. The privileging of content over form is implicit in his repeated insistence on 'direct emotional expression' as the subject-matter and method of modern dance.‡ But, by underlining the modernism of a fundamentally political and emotional form, Martin placed modern dance in a high art context. Kirstein,

on the other hand, despite the traditionally high art sources of classical ballet, positioned American ballet as 'low' by reinforcing its permeability with popular culture. My point is not only to show how unstable were the categories of legitimate and illegitimate – high and low – in American performance culture during the Depression, but also to show how the ballet/modern debate is, in fact, a screen for a dual critical practice of modernism.§

‡ These goals as Martin understood them were subsumed in his new coinage: 'metakinesis'. For further discussion of this theory in relation to ideology, see Franko 1997.

§ The genealogy of dance modernism, Susan Manning argues, has been disputed by critics along generic rather than philosophical lines. See Manning 1993.

Edna Ocko, the most articulate and prolific of left-wing dance critics, also evoked emotion as content to explain differences between formal classical and the new modern dancing:

> Notice how a decaying class of society, with nothing fresh and significant to say, encourages the creation of purely *formal* art, bereft of great feelings, incapable of stirring profound emotions. . . . On the other hand, the coming of age of a new class, sensing its potential strength, interested in expressing *its* ideas, determined to organize human feelings around its purposes, creates an art work rich in *content*, overflowing with human experience and understanding.
>
> (Ocko 1936: 26)

Equating 'human feelings' with content, as Ocko did, is a direct result of the form/content debate, one of whose variants was the ballet/modern debate. One consequence of this rhetoric, however, is that content was generally associated with the particular and form with the universal. Emotion tended to be located with content and abstraction with form. Furthermore, following this logic, emotion was the enemy of form.

What begs further understanding, however, is that radical performance practice used emotion as a conduit for, rather than as a vessel of, content. Emotion was neither unduly subjectified nor objectified but rather *transmitted*. It moved *between* people and thus was inappropriately anchored exclusively in either form or content (Figure 3).

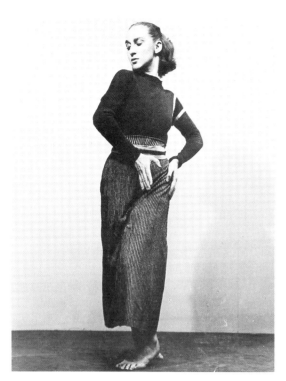

Figure 3: Anna Sokolow in an unidentified solo (1930s), Courtesy of the Dance Collection, New York Public Library for the Performing Arts at Lincoln Center, Astor, Lenox and Tilden Foundations

Funeral (1935). Unable to accuse Sokolow of a lack of professionalism, but clearly opposed to the choreographer's politics, Martin resorted to a theoretical argument impugning her decision to set the dance to a poem. His criticism focuses on the supposed incommensurabiltity of the poem as verbal artifact with the dance as non-verbal artifact. His argument bears examination because it sets down certain strictures about what dance can and cannot do, and raises the issue of abstraction as a fault of radical dance.

Martin's review of *Strange American Funeral* contains what is perhaps the most hard-bitten and transparent statement on the incommensurability of dance and language in the twentieth century:

> The great gulf that yawns between speech and movement is not easily bridged, for speech is essentially the means for expressing intellectualized experience, while movement is the more elemental stuff of the unintellectualized. The medium of words makes possible symbols of great economy, abstractions and generalizations; movement, being the direct externalization of emotional experience without the benefit of any rarefying processes, is extremely limited in the range of its symbolism and utterly incapable of abstraction and generalization.

(Martin 1935: 4)

Strange American Funeral provides a rare occasion in which Martin's philosophical concepts on dance are actively applied in his criticism. Not only are his critical tenets all exposed, but they are applied to one of the most celebrated left-wing choreographic works of the 1930s.* Sokolow used Michael Gold's poem about an employee's death in a steel mill

* *Strange American Funeral* premiered 9 June 1935 at the Park Circle Theater in New York as part of the New Dance League June Dance Festival. See Warren (1991: 302).

(Gold 1972: 126–8). Jan Clepak was the victim of an industrial accident – 'a worker who was caught in a flood of molten ore – whose flesh and blood turned to steel'.† Although the choreography of *Strange*

† Program from the dance recital of Anna Sokolow's Dance Unit, 28 February 1937. Anna Sokolow program file, Dance Collection, New York Public Library for the Performing Arts in New York City.

Without this interactive movement, the left itself considered emotion indulgent and moribund, labeling it 'bourgeois emotionalism', a term designating self-indulgent feelings that circulated only *inside* the individual, rather than from the individual to the social and back. In the same address, Ocko remarked:

> It is this faith, that true art can organize human feelings and emotions around profound social questions, that has brought forward a new trend in modern dance today,

(ibid.)

Ocko proposed that the world can be reorganized by dances that 'organize human feeling and emotions'. Elsewhere, she called revolutionary dances 'emotional crystallizations'. Martin might have agreed with her, except for the political context within which Ocko placed emotion.

Martin's most sustained attack on radical modern dance occurred on the occasion of the première of Anna Sokolow's *Strange American*

American Funeral is lost, critical accounts indicate that Sokolow eschewed realism for a montage of images concerning life and death in relation to metallization and humanity. Martin's review indicates that the choreography took a variety of standpoints in time and space. As in Gold's poem 'Strange funeral in Braddock', Clepak appears and reappears in flashbacks. Clearly, Sokolow relied in this work on the poetic rather than narrative dimensions of dance composition, one important element of which was the choreographic rendering of a change from flesh and blood to steel. Muriel Rukeyser's review in *New Theatre* (July 1935) indicated that the motif of metallized bodies was a recurrent image: 'The solid steel block of dancers, locked at the elbows . . . fixed the meaning of the dance' (Graff 1997: 69).*

Because the text was recited in performance – it had already been set to music by Elie Siegmeister – Sokolow's choreography did not meet Martin's criterion for modern dance as 'the direct externalization of emotional experience'. Martin accused Sokolow of confusing danced content with linguistic abstraction. In reality, his objection was to the contextualization and social situatedness of her emotion: 'It was evident', Martin wrote, 'that Miss Sokolow had been deeply moved by the poem. Many individual passages of her composition were superb not only in their integrity of feeling but in their boldness of imagination. But the dance as a whole was inchoate and pointless' (Martin 1935: 4). Emotion and abstraction are opposed in Martin's thinking because emotion is direct and unmediated whereas abstraction is formal and symbolic.†

Sokolow's emotion in *Strange American Funeral* was mediated by her social surroundings, and thus contravened Martin's requirement that the particular in art be so by virtue of its origin in the private. Accusing Sokolow of abstraction for rendering emotion social seems terminologically perverse except for the fact that the onus of the critique was placed on the articulation of poetic language during the dance. This choice of pretext for criticism was an ideological smoke-screen.

Martin wrote another essay on Sokolow and modern dance in 1939. Here, the radical choreographer is introduced in exemplary terms: 'Of all the dancers who have associated themselves with the political Left, none has made clearer his intentions as an artist than Anna Sokolow' (Martin 1939: 8). In recognizing Sokolow as an exemplar of a people's dance art, however, Martin defines radical dance as the heir to nineteenth-century romanticism, which is 'nothing more nor less, indeed, in its historical origins, than a people's art' (ibid.). Martin posits three criteria of romantic art making it also a people's art: 'the movement must be vernacular movement . . . the subject matter must be free in its imaginative range . . . it must be entirely innocent of arbitrary formalism' (ibid.). By imaginative range, Martin means 'a freeing of the passions to re-experience or to enjoy synthetically high moments of feeling or excitement' (ibid.). Martin does not ascribe these characteristics to Sokolow alone:

> The entire modern dance, indeed, is perhaps the most striking example of true romanticism in our time, and Miss Sokolow's approach is only a slightly more 'class conscious' aspect of it. To look at the essential character of romance in its historic beginnings must give to the modern dance a clear notion of its own antiquity, its basic logic, and, above all, its future methods of procedure.
>
> (ibid.)

Likening a 'people's art' – that is, an art for and about the proletarian masses – to romanticism is a way to evacuate the historical specificity of radical modern dance, as well as to blur distinctions between modernism and radicalism (or bourgeois and revolutionary dance). Martin gives Sokolow a leading place in the modern dance movement at the

* Since Sokolow also choreographed works on Italian fascism during the 1930s – particularly *Excerpts from a War Poem (F. T. Marinetti)* – it is possible that fascism and capitalism came in for parallel critiques in *Strange American Funeral*. On metallization in fascist performance, see Schnapp 1996.

† It is tempting to read Martin's review as a critical quid pro quo for left-wing critiques of Graham as cold, passionless and abstract. Martin turns these same accusations against Sokolow, the most accomplished of the politically radical choreographers. On the debate over Graham's relation to emotion and coldness, see 'Emotivist movement and histories of modernism: the case of Martha Graham' in Franko 1995: 38–74.

price of a theory that de-politicizes her dances. This theory has the particular advantage of reinforcing Martin's earlier position on abstraction as inimical to emotional expression:

> The sole function of form in a simple and natural art of this sort is to insure that the material makes sense. Obviously this is more difficult than to build a synthetic makeshift to titillate the esthete, for it demands roots in life. . . . The spoken word, that final admission of failure, cannot illuminate movement, it can only render it unnecessary.
>
> (ibid.)

In a 1938 essay on dance and abstraction Martin reintegrates the necessity for an abstraction consonant with dance modernism. He gives two alternative definitions of abstraction in dance. The first 'is that approach to the dance which puts aside all dramatic and literary program, and deals exclusively in terms of movement, without what is generally referred to as meaning' (Martin, 1938: n.p.). As an example of this kind of abstraction – one totally devoid of 'dramatic program', but also of 'social content' – Martin cites the Rockettes: 'as complete abstraction as it is possible for the human body to attain' (ibid.)* (Figure 4). But he also speaks of the ability of dance to convey 'emotional experience' as abstraction: 'It [dance] is the medium for conveying those concepts which are

* Martin was not the first to make such a judgement. See Kracauer's 'The mass ornament' (1929) (1995: 75–88). In Kracauer, the kickline's abstraction is the aesthetic equivalent of instrumental rationality. This layering of aesthetic and ideological analysis is absent from Martin's writing. For further analysis in the spirit of Kracauer, see Jelavich 1993: 180-6.

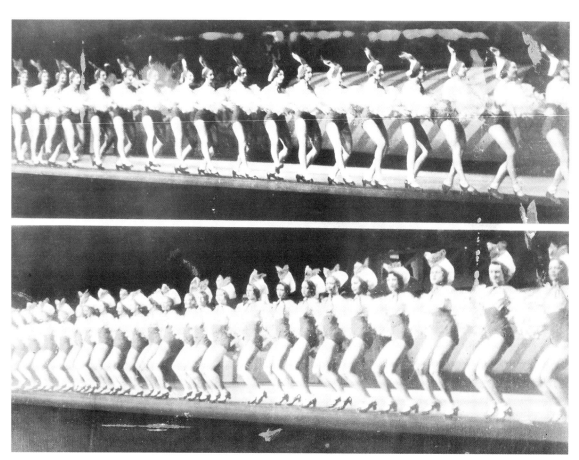

Figure 4: The Rockettes chorus line in the 1930s. Courtesy of the Dance Collection, New York Public Library for the Performing Arts at Lincoln Center, Astor, Lenox and Tilden Foundations

still too deeply rooted in emotional experience to be objectified in factual [understand: linguistic?] terms' (ibid.). Using music as an example, Martin asserts: 'we are inclined to demand an elevated impersonality of emotion, and from the dancer we have every reason to ask the same. . . . Without this process of abstraction he is bound to be unintelligible.' Through the issue of movement's intelligibility, Martin posits the necessity for abstraction in dance. If one compares the 1939 article on romanticism with the 1938 article on abstraction, their concerns converge around this term. Of a people's art, Martin wrote:

> Movement which is readily communicative to all men must be essentially that which all men employ in their own day-by-day living. If it is heightened beyond the ability of all men to perform, as it must be for purposes of art to make it more vivid, it must still remain emotionally recognizable. When it is altered beyond this point, either by deliberate manipulation or by unconscious mechanicalization, it is dead material.

> (ibid.)

In the article on abstraction, however, intelligibility is removed from day-by-day terms because the emotional experience of modern dance cannot be 'objectified in factual terms' (ibid.). In the context of this argument, however, 'factual' is glossed as 'literal' as well as 'literary' and associated with discursive rather than movement practices. Clearly, Martin is balancing two utterly opposed conceptions of abstraction: as universalized meaning and as pure form. He does not believe that modern dance is modernist precisely because he cannot conceive that universalized meaning might be conveyed in 'pure' form. Above all, abstraction is a theoretical escape hatch for Martin; but one that leads him dangerously close to absurdity.

Let us return for a moment to Martin's review of Sokolow's *Strange American Funeral*. What is 'elevated impersonality of emotion' if not 'a symbol of great economy'? Such a symbol, however, was what Martin reproached Sokolow for essaying in *Strange American Funeral*. Rather than focus on the symbol, however, he focused on Gold's poem as

purveyor of symbols in contrast to which movement was 'the *direct* externalization of emotional experience' (Martin 1935: 4; my emphasis). The 'rarefying process' that Martin denied to Sokolow's choreography in the review is difficult to distinguish from the universalization of the particular that Martin allows modern dance in general. In a dance of social significance that makes no attempt to abstract its subject-matter beyond avoiding literalism, Martin proclaims 'dance is utterly incapable of abstraction and generalization'. In a dance, that of the Rockettes, which proposes the endless circulation of capital as sex, Martin sees 'complete abstraction', and for other modern dance that feigns to avoid the ideological split between capital and labor, Martin sees that 'the process of abstraction' ensures intelligibility through 'elevated impersonality'. He defends the primacy of feeling in the 1930s, but cuts feeling off from any politics.

III

The most successful realization of Kirstein's theory of Americanized ballet was Lew Christensen's *Filling Station* (1938).* The main character is ostensibly proletarian, because the ballet, according to Kirstein, was 'about work, today'. 'It couldn't be put in a factory,' he adds, 'on an open road or on a farm, because we didn't have enough dancers to suggest a mass of workers' [262]. Mac, the Filling Station Attendant, was, nevertheless, 'the type of self-reliant, agreeable and frank American working-man' [263] (Figure 5). Mac's opening variation is virtuosic, signaling, in Kirstein's terms, his 'brilliant resourcefulness' as a worker (ibid.). His filling station is then visited by two truck drivers, Roy and Ray, who are presented as 'tumblers' and 'vaudeville knock-about comedians' (ibid.). They are succeeded by a humdrum bourgeois couple: the Motorist ('a combination of Casper Milquetoast and Mut'), his Wife ('green-blond hair, summer slacks and sinister

* *Filling Station*, which Kirstein commissioned and authored, was premiered by Ballet Caravan at Avery Memorial Auditorium, Hartford, Connecticut, on 6 January 1938, on a program of 'all-American ballets'. It was revived in 1951 by the San Francisco Ballet where Christensen eventually settled. It is being revived again by the same company in the year of this writing.

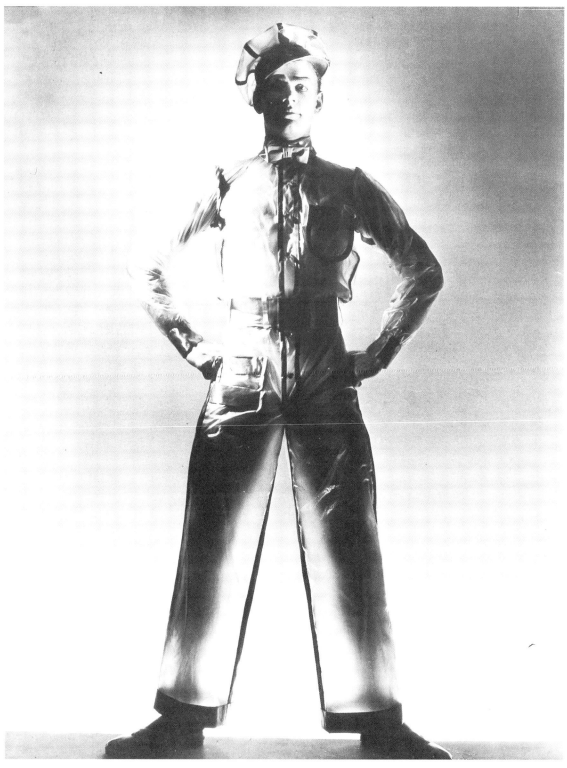

Figure 5: Lew Christensen as Mac in *The Filling Station*, 1938. Photo: George Platt Lynes, courtesy of the photographer's estate

green celluloid-visor') and their little girl ('a nightmare twin of Shirley Temple or Little Orphan Annie') (ibid.). The Child's toe-work 'was indicated as the prize-number of a spoiled child's dancing-class graduation exercises' (ibid.). They are followed by a Rich Girl and a Rich Boy who dance drunk until a gangster intrudes on the scene to hold them up. *Filling Station* was populated by balletic versions of the lower, middle and upper classes, cartoon-like figures on to all of whose movement characteristics classical vocabulary was 'grafted'.* Kirstein opined that *Filling Station* combined 'American social humor' with 'international theatrical dancing' [265]. If classical dance could be so readily grafted on to popular culture figures many of whom were derived from the funny papers, vaudeville and the Follies, Kirstein was positioning classical ballet alongside the entertainment industry aesthetic just as modern dance was positioned alongside the labor movement aesthetic.

* 'The traditional classic dance was grafted on American character-dancing.' Kirstein 1937: 264.

But, given the oppositional relationship between labor and popular culture in the 1930s, the labor theme Kirstein foregrounded in *Filling Station* was right-wing. Publicity for the ballet shows its lack of connection to any concern for the working class. Although Mac is a worker, he is hardly a militant worker. The program note for the world première states that the ballet is 'about an ordinary working man who does his job whatever the circumstances'.† This worker, who could have issued from the pages of a government report on optimal employee disposition, was a *danseur noble* (Lew Christensen). Mac holds the (empty) place of a prince in a poetics of the ordinary. Publicity for the work hedges on this thematic innovation by explaining how the ballet re-exoticizes everyday life:

† *Filling Station* program, the Christensen–Caccialanza Collection, the San Francisco Performing Arts Library and Museum.

> Some everyday happenings and objects need only be surprised out of their daily context by transformation into terms of the stage to lose their banality, suddenly to

become more exotic than India and almost as strange as another planet.‡

‡ The Ballet Caravan publicity sheet, the Christensen–Caccialanza Collection, the San Francisco Performing Arts Library and Museum.

This return of the exotic in the ordinary hardly seems to fulfill Kirstein's program of ballet modernism as 'living expression of the immediate' (Kirstein 1935: 22) able to establish ballet 'in the service of the greatest mass public' (ibid.: 20).

Filling Station presented a danced portrayal of the American worker's character as open, frank and agreeable, and thus unlike foreign working-class elements in urban America. There is an implication, as well, that in his simple elegance, Mac must avoid any over-intellectualization familiar in foreign and politicized elements. The denizens of Kirstein's pastoral/industrial landscape 'have an unspoiled, American, rather athletic quality that is pleasant' (Denby 1986: 48). *Filling Station* allowed associations with character dance traditions to introduce class distinctions in a ballet composition (as well they might in almost any classical ballet scenario) but eliminated the ethnic positions which gave class positions meaning. Thus Mac, the worker, could be both familiar and unfamiliar – the secret of his 'agreeableness'. The worker was a ballet star surrounded by music-hall exotics. What *Filling Station* exoticized was class itself as a social issue, submerging its edge in the familiarly humorous references of mediatized popular culture. Kirstein's equality of the popular with the exotic is as absurd from the point of view of his stated intentions as is Martin's equality of politically engaged art with abstraction.§ These improbable whirligigs are moments of truth – rhetorical moments where dance modernism encounters the specter of social engagement.

§ Although the influence of Jean Cocteau's ideas on the poetics of the ordinary is clearly present here, the ideas also clash with the socio-cultural context of Depression America.

IV

Both Kirstein and Martin engaged in conceptual double-binds that erected modernism at the sites of popular and mass culture, respectively. Both saw dance as the process of an abstraction of politics from movement. Both, in short, were ideologues of aesthetic modernism. Kirstein moves ostensibly from high to low, but aestheticizes low as what he considers to be the timeless technical system of ballet classicism, an enduring abstraction of human movement. Martin moves ostensibly from low to high by depersonalizing or privatizing emotion as both universal and direct, and thus acting to remove the social impetus from its manifestations in dancing bodies.

Despite their shared ideological goals, there is only one point at which the arguments of these two critics form a rhetorical tangent: when Martin attributes to the Rockette the qualities of abstraction proper to Kirstein's ballet dancer. It seems here that Martin, perhaps unwittingly, confirms the hidden ties between ballet and commercial theater. The Rockettes personified 'complete abstraction'. The culture war between modern dance and classical ballet represented by these two seminal figures is turned on its head by this identification of the Rockettes' kickline with aesthetic abstraction. Granted, his observation was made in passing and never enshrined in one of Martin's books; but it is a slip revealing that the ballet–modern wars were an ideological screen, one of whose long-term effects has been to eradicate radical performance from living memory.

Since neither ballet nor modern was situated unequivocally as 'high' or 'low', any historically informed comparison between them raises issues of class in relation to performance. Ballet maintained its 'high' status by appearing to be 'low' (popular), and radical modern dance was perceived as 'high' by deprecating the commodifications of popular culture in favor of the working-class audience. Each contained the supplement of the other, a supplementarity within the identity of each genre embodied by the repressed figure of the chorus girl who was both an ersatz or would-be ballet dancer and a proletarian entertainment industry worker. By associating herself with a ballet aesthetic, the chorus girl enabled classical dance to merge with

popular culture; by representing the antithesis of modern dance seriousness through her sexiness and commercialism, she made radical modern dance appear to be an elitist project. The chorus girl was, in short, the dangerous supplement of American theatrical dancing. She shows that dance is labor since she sold her labor for a wage, but she also implicitly states that woman's work is sex. By substituting emotion for sex the modern dancer implicitly proposes her labor of movement be considered as potential lodged in the person rather than a demeaning activity affirming the spectator's sexual titillation. It was difficult to assess the modern dancer's activity with respect to its exchange value. As Martin's theory demonstrated, a viewer of modern dance should discover the dancer's emotivo-physical patterning in himself as an equally personal and thus unexchangeable experience. The separation of modern dance from the market was ideologically reassuring to those who opposed the dominant culture (the modern dancer could never or only rarely earn a wage), but conceptually troubling to others because of its visual evidence for labor potential whose value eluded market calculations. In other words, in its very means of communication, historical modern dance contradicted the notion of labor as a commodity, replacing it with that of the dancer as producer.* Her labor of emotion in the body productive of a once radical ideology is, when reconstructed today, what makes crowds roar.

* Although I adapt this phrase from Walter Benjamin's essay on Bertolt Brecht, 'The author as producer', I do not mean production in their sense as an artistic equivalent for technology. Quite to the contrary, the American modern dancer produces revolution as a bodily and emotional phenomenon rather than a critical, and therefore scientific, one. See Benjamin 1977.

REFERENCES

Benjamin, Walter (1977) 'The author as producer', in his *Understanding Brecht*, trans. Anna Bostock, London: Verso, pp. 85-104.
Choreography by George Balanchine. A Catalogue of Works (1983), New York: Eakins Press Foundation.
Conner, Lynne (1997) *Spreading the Gospel of Modern Dance: Newspaper Dance Criticism in the United*

States, 1850–1934, Pittsburgh, PA: University of Pittsburgh Press.

Denby, Edwin (1986) *Dance Writings*, ed. Robert Cornfield and William McKay, New York: Alfred A. Knopf.

Francisco, Charles (1979) *The Radio City Music Hall: An Affectionate History*, New York: E. P. Dutton.

Franko, Mark (1995) *Dancing Modernism/Performing Politics*, Bloomington: Indiana University Press.

Franko, Mark (1996) 'History/theory – criticism/practice', in Susan Leigh Foster (ed.) *Corporealities: Dancing, Knowledge, Culture and Power*, London: Routledge, pp. 25–52.

Franko, Mark (1997) 'Nation, class, and ethnicities in modern dance of the 1930s', *Theatre Journal* 49: 475–91.

Gold, Michael (1972) 'Strange funeral in Braddock', in *Mike Gold: A Literary Anthology*, ed. Michael Folsom, New York: International Publishers, pp. 126–8.

Graff, Ellen (1997) *Stepping Left. Dance and Politics in New York City, 1928–1942*, Durham, NC: Duke University Press.

Hardy, Camille (1980) 'Ballet girls and broilers: the development of the American chorus girl, 1895–1919', *Ballet Review* 8(1): 96–127.

Horwitz, Dawn Lille (1985) 'Fokine and the American musical', *Ballet Review* 13(2) (Summer): 57–72.

Jelavich, Peter (1993) *Berlin Cabaret*, Cambridge, MA: Harvard University Press.

Kirstein, Lincoln (1934) 'Revolutionary ballet forms', *New Theatre* (October): 12–14.

Kirstein, Lincoln (1935) 'The dance as theatre', *New Theatre* (May): 20–2.

Kirstein, Lincoln (1937) 'Blast at ballet', in *Ballet: Bias and Belief. Three Pamphlets Collected and Other Dance Writings of Lincoln Kirstein*, New York: Dance Horizons, 1963, p. 246.

Kirstein, Lincoln (1963) *Ballet: Bias and Belief. Three Pamphlets Collected and Other Dance Writings of Lincoln Kirstein*, New York: Dance Horizons.

Kracauer, Siegfried (1995 [1929]) 'The mass ornament', in his *The Mass Ornament: Weimar Essays*, ed. and trans. Thomas Y. Levin, Cambridge, MA: Harvard University Press, pp. 75–88.

Levine, Lawrence L. (1988) *Highbrow/Lowbrow: the Emergence of Cultural Hierarchy in America*, Cambridge, MA: Harvard University Press.

MacAloon, John J. (1984) 'Olympic Games and the theory of spectacle in modern societies', in *Rite. Drama, Festival, Spectacle. Rehearsals toward a Theory of Cultural Performance*, ed. John J. MacAloon, Philadelphia, PA: ISHI, pp. 241–80.

Manning, Susan (1993) *Ecstasy and the Demon: Feminism and Nationalism in the Dances of Mary Wigman*, Berkeley and Los Angeles: University of California Press.

Martin, John (1935) 'The dance: with words. Anna Sokolow ventures a choreographic setting for a new poem', *The New York Times* (30 June): 4.

Martin, John (1938) 'The dance: abstraction. Staring the hobgoblin out of countenance', *The New York Times* (11 December).

Martin, John (1939) 'The dance: Romanticism. A venerable tradition with light to shed on modern trends', *The New York Times* (5 March): 8.

Ocko, Edna (1934) 'The revolutionary dance movement', *New Theatre* (June): 27–8; reprinted in Franko (1995: 125).

Ocko, Edna (1936) 'Dance in a changing world: a new trend', in *The Proceedings of the First National Dance Congress and Festival*, New York.

Ocko, Edna (1994) 'Reviewing on the left: the dance criticism of Edna Ocko', in 'Of, By, and For the People: Dancing on the Left in the 1930s', an issue of *Studies in Dance History* 5: 65–103.

Schnapp, Jeffrey T. (1996) *Staging Fascism: 18BL and the Theater of Masses for Masses*, Stanford, CA: Stanford University Press.

Turner, Victor (1995) *The Ritual Process: Structure and Anti-Structure*, New York: Walter de Gruyter.

Waring, James (1967) 'Five essays on dancing', *Ballet Review* 2(1): 65–77.

Warren, Larry (1991) *Anna Sokolow: the Rebellious Spirit*, Princeton, NJ: Dance Horizons.

I Never Go Anywhere I Can't Drive Myself

Leslie Hill and Helen Paris

LESLIE HILL

Can you really 'perform' on the internet? Considering that futurists predict that the most profound shift to occur in the twenty-first century will be the shift from a place-oriented to a 'placeless' society, this is something I want to know. As we conduct more and more of our communication, research and commerce on-line and as the world around us shifts from analog to digital, physical location becomes less and less of a determining factor in our ability to do our work, access information, keep in touch with friends and buy or sell. Having an email account, internet access and a computer, of course, become increasingly important to our ability to function as members of a community, to interact with our peers, to access and to make work. What does this mean for performance? It's one thing to publish text on the internet, but how can one conceptually, atmospherically and emotively make the leap from atoms to electronic bits when it comes to Annie Sprinkle's cervix? Scan the cervix, upload it and program it to blink on and off, create some roll-over text, embed an element of inter-activity for the audience, forge hot-button links to other cervix-related sites? No doubt people would then say things like, 'I went to Annie Sprinkle's cervix last night', because people tend to talk about sites they have down-loaded as places they have 'been'.* This is interesting because film and television provide infinitely more sophisticated audio-visual experiences of locations, but a person who watches a documentary film about the magnetic pole doesn't say, 'I went to the magnetic pole last night', whereas with web sites, which are comparatively slow and clunky, people do talk in terms of places they have 'been' or 'visited', or are 'going' to.

These musings bring me back again and again to Walter Benjamin's observation that the contextual integration of art in tradition found its expression in the cult, and that 'even the most perfect reproduction of a

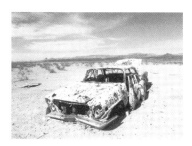

Junk car, Route 66, 1998. Photo; Hill/Paris

* Since writing this I have found that indeed Annie Sprinkle's cervix is on-line and may be visited at: *http://www.heck.com/annie/cervix-main.html* – with a special message from Annie herself, 'Dear Online Explorer, Welcome to my intervaginal superhighway, where the wonderful world of cervix awaits you . . .'

Performance Research 3(2), pp.102–108 © Routledge 1998

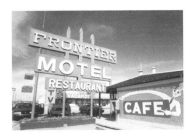

Frontier, Route 66, 1998. Photo: Hill/Paris

work of art is lacking in one element: its presence in time and space, its unique existence in the place where it happens to be' (Benjamin 1969: 220). As a performer working in real-space, real-time situations, I was able to maintain, at least in my own mind, a smug distance from the diluting implications of 'The work of art in the age of mechanical reproduction'. Performance, more than any other art form, has retained its connection to 'the cult', existing fleetingly in the times and places of the performances, which is what gives it much of its power and also makes it notoriously difficult to document and, let's face it, nearly impossible to make a living at. Anyway, coming from the 'cultish' world of performance, I have been intrigued by the notion of the world-wide web and the idea of people 'going' to all these places, and it gives me pause for thought as a maker, when I try and work out the relationship of place and authenticity on the net: is art that exists only within cyber-space an original that has transcended the need for reproduction or is it a simulation that supersedes the need for the existence of an 'authentic' original?

Helen Paris and I decided to make a web piece that would explore notions of place and placelessness in performance and so in terms of form and content the piece had to be devised around real-space, real-time experiences with specific individuals and virtual ones, uploaded for access by a potentially limitless, but strangely invisible, audience. The genre of the road trip is at once totally specific, totally place-orien-tated and yet intrinsically fluid as scenery morphs gradually from city to country, from mountain to plain. We decided to locate our perform-ance within the genre of the road trip, performing a time-based piece simultaneously on two-lane byways and the 'info-superhighway'. The venue for our performance was, then, the 'real' space of Route 66, the first American Highway to link East to West, running from Chicago to LA, and the virtual space of the road trip site: *http://www.edutv.org/drive/billboard.html* As the performers, we acted as linchpins between the two venues, between place and placelessness, between real and virtual. In making a piece using new technology we wanted to ask new questions about our practice, and also to make work in a unique way. If we were treating the internet as a venue for performance we wanted to use it to do things that no other venue could do and this linking of place and placelessness, of site-specific and cyberspatial, seemed, to us, to fit the bill. Out on the old highway the sites are more site-specific – there are no Starbucks or Café Dome, no chains, no nationalized adver-tising logos, but the epic semiotics of roadside cafés announced by giant astronauts, flashing neon rockets, spinning rooftop hamburgers and ice-cream cones, the four-storey hot-dog man and hand-painted barn-side announcements. The places are run by mom and pop owners, not multinationals, and no two places are the same. By self-publishing stories and photographs daily during the course of our month-long trip

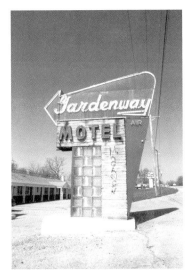

Gardenway, Route 66, 1998. Photo: Hill/Paris

from Chicago to LA and back again, we were able to link the placeless realm of cyberspace to such site-specific venues as Dixie Lee Evans' Exotic World Museum and retired strippers' ranch,* communicating a real-space, real-time project into a globally accessible venue with a 'live' or time-based

* Recently immortalized on canvas by Sadie Lee in her 1997 National Portrait Gallery exhibition, sponsored by the **BP** Travel Award.

dimension expressed in the daily evolution of the virtual journey in tandem with the physical journey. In this simultaneous negotiation of old and new highways, we felt we were expanding, rather than diminishing, our practice as performers and maintaining, rather than rejecting, the 'cult' status of live work.

All roads lead to Baudrillard and ours is no different. Baudrillard cites the most important event of modern history as the disappearance of 'the real', as the late twentieth century becomes a world of social and technological transparencies and simulacra. In his book *The Perfect Crime*, Baudrillard investigates the murder of reality, detective fashion, using traces of evidence, marks of imperfection, to unravel the crime. In his work he poses the artist as one of the primary sources of evidence, of imperfection, of traces of reality:

> The artist, too, is always close to committing the perfect crime: saying nothing. But he turns away from it, and his work is the trace of that criminal imperfection. The artist is, in Michaux's words, the one who, with all his might, resists the fundamental drive not to leave traces.

(Baudrillard 1996: 1)

As well as negotiating the performer's relationship to place and placelessness, Helen and I were interested in exploring how artists might translate 'evidence' from the real to the virtual, how they might mark their passing in either realm. How does one leave a cigarette in the ashtray in cyberspace? Before we left England we began compiling an extensive, eclectic archive including video-taped messages from site-specific English locations, such as Derek Jarman's garden or the tomb of Karl Marx; old maps of Shropshire and Skye; family photographs and recipes; seed packets of English primroses and cowslips; souvenirs from the Tower of London; 'original' Sherlock Holmes memorabilia from Baker Street; Sainsburys digestive biscuits and Red Label tea; tape-recorded and written narratives, and of course, the BBC Radio 4 'Shipping Forecast' and 'Gardeners' Question Time' . Our idea was to leave a trail of evidence, of literal and metaphorical messages in bottles, in our wake as we travelled and conversely to replace our existing archive with a new archive collected *en route* from the people and places we encountered. Discovered randomly in isolation from each other by people along Route 66, our stories, objects and images were at once fragmentary narratives and links in the long thin chain of a much larger piece, connected by our physical presence as we travelled and

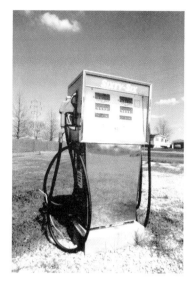

Gas pump, Route 66, 1998. Photo: Hill/Paris

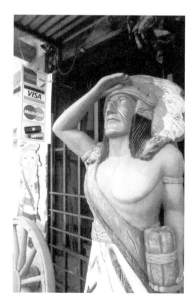

Indian salutes, Route 66, 1998. Photo: Hill/Paris

simultaneously by the creation of the time-based web site which offered accounts of both evidence left behind and evidence gathered. The only full account of the piece, of course, lives in our personal experiences, but next to that, the web site provides the most cohesive account of the project through our daily journals, our 'messages in bottles' and the photographic histories of lemon curd left on doorsteps or seeds planted by the roadside. The self-conscious fragmentation of the narrative and of the trail of evidence collected and left behind, and the non-linear possibilities of the web site worked for me, at any rate, to create a mode of performance that was able to use multimedia and telecommunications within a format that was symbiotic in relation to the content of the piece. The virtual was grounded in the real. Real space, real time lead the project and we felt uncompromised, in this case, as 'live artists'. Performance sensibility and the juxtaposition between going places and 'going places' worked to create performance in a new way, for new audiences, stretching, rather than cutting loose, our tether to the unique cult status of performance.

HELEN PARIS

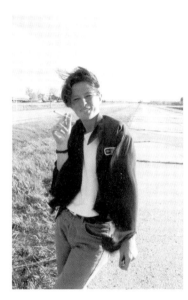

Helen Paris smokes, Route 66, 1998. Photo: Hill/Paris

Contact and communication are the mainstays of performance in my book, and as Route 66 was the first road in the USA to link people from East to West and the world-wide web is the single greatest communication enabler the world has yet seen, together they seemed to provide an ideal 'venue' for our live art road trip as we drove the 4,456 miles from Chicago to LA and back again, both literally, via a red Pontiac Grand-Am, and 'cyberspatially', via a daily updated web site. I was pretty excited about this project, because a good venue is hard to find. Always avoiding the trap of making funding-led work, the logistics of the fiscal arrangements demanded by such a venture were instantly lost under a pile of fat notebooks Leslie and I sent to each other between London and Dublin, full of discussions of the epic Great Wall of China crossing by Marina Abramovic and Ulay; Jack Kerouac's six-month stint on Desolation Peak; Laurie Anderson's spontaneous hitchhike to the North Pole; and details of how we would cook tins of beans off the car engine. For this project we distilled the elements of performance to the relationship between the performer and the audience based on the simple concepts of 'give' and 'take', determining that we would make these elements tangible by literally giving/leaving elements of the familiar from our own lives in the form of stories, photographs, letters and videotapes, in exchange for stories, recipes, snapshots and artifacts collected *en route*. Embracing the dynamic of tourism inherent in the project, we incorporated quintessentially 'British' items into our 'give' archive (Rough Scottish Oatcakes and whiskey, an authentically yellowed map of Sherlock Holmes's London, the Tower of London 'Steal the Crown Jewels' board game, etc.) and collected Route 66 memorabilia in return (a St Louis Arch snowball scene, gasoline pump salt and pepper shakers, tequila lollipops, etc.). We packed our 'give' archive into a large suitcase, then planted a gold star on the 'Begin Route 66' signpost in Adams Street, Chicago and we were off . . . or 'on'. . . . Instantly I was filled with performance anxiety. What if no one comes?

Initially we had no way of knowing who would attend our three-week performance, either virtually or in the flesh. The chat page on the web site enabling our virtual audience to leave comments was a *tabula rasa*, as were the rolls of film and the audio- and videotape we had for documenting the 'real' audience of Route 66; and then of course the rehearsal is never the same experience as the performance. . . . First off I just didn't look right. An advocate of minimalism; the sight of myself walking towards a tiny café in the middle of nowhere armed with a video camera, digital camera, DAT machine, microphone, 35mm camera and large suitcase did not fit into my vision of making a profound visceral or emotive, honest and meaningful contact with an audience (let alone lead me to think I was embodying the keen, honed outline of the lonesome traveller). Marina Abramovic, however, describes the Great Wall of China crossing as her ideal journey, when nothing is fixed, because this is where she found the 'edge that makes you wake' (Abramovic 1993: 46) and as I entered the Midway Café, Adrian, Texas, it soon became clear that the type of interaction possible in this project had a spontaneity and life of its own. The café, like most others on the now decommissioned route, was pretty empty. Mostly it contained a few regulars, one, a man in his mid-70s whom I heard the waitress call Bob, was sitting at the counter reading the paper, a bright green visor perched on his shock of white hair. Little did I know that only a short while later we would be 2 miles up the road following Bob's old red pickup truck as he led us to his farm where we were introduced to Ronnie Jackson and given the guided tour of their collection of eight crop-spraying planes. 'Me and Ronnie made this here one without even a plan to follow,' stated Bob proudly, pointing to a fine yellow model. 'It took a lot of beer.' It appeared that the bigger and more complicated the plane, the larger the quantity of beer involved in production; so much so, that part of Bob's tour included a visit to the 'hangover room'.

The contact with the virtual audience had its own unique dynamism. The web site made the project about the specific and the infinite at the same time; the potential to make contact with one waitress in a diner in the middle of the Mojave Desert and simultaneously with the rest of the world. Getting lost on the road one day as it eluded us for a moment, we stopped in a quiet street to ask directions. The street was just a few houses really, in the middle of the vast expanse of Oklahoma plains. It was early morning but an old woman in a bright red dressing

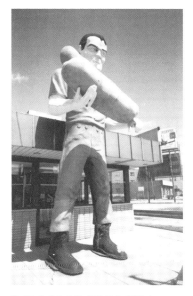

Giant dog (hot), Route 66, 1998. Photo: Hill/Paris

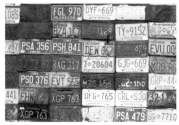

Licence plates, Route 66, 1998. Photo: Hill/Paris

106

gown was out getting her mail from the box at the end of her garden. Despite the early hour she was perfectly made up, her lipstick matching her gown, and holding a half-eaten, fleshy avocado in her hand. As we drove off, I turned back and watched her getting smaller and smaller until she was just a tiny red dot in all that landscape and I thought about how later I would be sending that information about her housecoat out into the other vast landscape of cyberspace. As detailed and honest a performance as I might give in the flesh. Not to say the conveyance of this material was seamless; a cantankerous HTML code, a temperamental connection cable for the digital camera and an inability to get on-line any time before 2.00 a.m. (Route 66 may have been decommissioned and deserted but the cyberspatial highway was one big traffic jam) led to a level of tension never experienced in performance nerves. Updated every few hours, our performance on the site engendered remarkably similar feelings to live performance, high pressure and high adrenalin. In live performance, however, there is always the reassuring certainty that if you make a mistake, you are likely to be the only one to be aware of it. Here in our virtual venue, one missed-out dot or a misplaced '<' could render communication with the audience impossible, and the presence of our virtual audience was a constant one, even when they were absent, so to speak.

When we picnicked in the desert on an old disused part of the road in the hot Californian sun just before the end of our trip from East to West I knew I would be posting the exact details of the meal, the hot smell of the desert and the euphoria of having got thus far, on to the web that evening. Our virtual audience left evidence of their participation not only in comments on the web site chat page but through posting actual requests, such as one very specific entreaty for a recipe for pecan pie, to be written by a waitress in a diner on to her order pad. Our real-life actions became informed by the virtual audience and thus made me wonder exactly who was the performer and who the audience.

In Truxston, Arizona, we met Mildred who had run the Frontier Café and Motel together with her husband for twenty-seven years. Since he died in 1990, she hadn't known what to do as regards the business: 'I'm 69–70 this year – and I know I should give it up, but I always think ... "You never know who you might meet tomorrow."' Mildred's philosophy became a sort of motto of our journey, the 'here and now dynamic' when potentially anything could happen on our performance-in-motion with its ever changing audience. I was still questioning the ownership of performer/audience roles when we met Dixie Lee Evans at Exotic World, Wild Road. Dixie led us round her museum of strip-tease, informing us that Aristophanes was the founder of burlesque and in the next moment, pointing to a large golden urn amidst the boas and *diamanté* G-strings, crying: 'That's Sherri Champagne! Now she just wouldn't wear any costume that didn't have

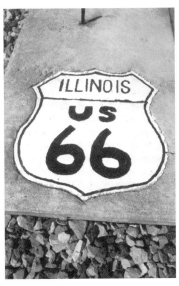

Sidewalk, Route 66, 1998. Photo: Hill/Paris

the picture of a champagne glass on it.' At times, framed in a doorway, Dixie would hold out her arms dramatically and state: 'We took what was real and we exaggerated it, we made it larger than life . . . That was burlesque.' What, we wondered, was our relationship to the real? We took what was real and made it digital, in stories and photographs from the unforgettable residents of Route 66, formatted for viewing on a web site that remains 'live' even after the journey is over. In return we left the evidence of our journey in hand-written messages in bottles; in audio-taped stories of where we came from; in Polaroids of ourselves on location; in a trail of seeds planted from Chicago to LA; in a box of mint imperials in the Baghdad Café, the final oasis before entering the Mojave Desert; in video footage of Karl Marx's grave in Highgate Cemetery atop Abe Lincoln's tomb in Springfield; in a fuzzy felt raven finger-puppet from the Tower of London in the belly of a giant blue whale at an Oklahoma swimming hole; and in a tiny beefeater statue left on a red and white table-cloth in a diner in Illinois. These traces we left for future audiences who would pick up the trail. All of these markers, digital and atomic, are still out there in the vastness of cyber-space and the old American highway.

Following on from their on-line Route 66 road trip through two-lane byways and info-superhighways, artists Leslie Hill and Helen Paris abandon their bright red sports car for a table at 'Les Deux Magots', the sidewalk café at the heart of the Parisian Left Bank writers' culture once frequented by authors such as Hemingway and Stein. From their stationary position, watching the world go by, Hill and Paris make fresh explorations of the significance of 'place' in a world where more and more of our daily contact occurs in the 'placeless' realm of cyberspace, and muse on the past, present and future of the great love affair between writers and cafés. Why does the solitary act of writing crave the public forum of the café? How do we form communities and identities on-line as opposed to in the flesh? Please visit the new site, now up at *http://www.leftbank.org*

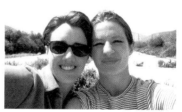

Leslie Hill picnics, Route 66, 1998. Photo: Hill/Paris

REFERENCES:

Abramovic, Marina (1993) 'A great wall', in C. Carr (ed.) *On Edge: Performance at the End of the Twentieth Century*, Middletown, CT: Wesleyan University Press.

Baudrillard, Jean (1996) *The Perfect Crime*, London: Verso.

Benjamin, Walter (1969) The work of art in the age of mechanical reproduction', in his *Illuminations: Essays and Reflections*, ed. Hannah Arendt, trans. Harry Zohn, New York: Schocken.

Leslie Hill and Helen Paris, Route 66, 1998. Photo: Hill/Paris

Backwords: 1,293 Steps

Space is a practiced place.

(Michel de Certeau 1984: 117)

If one wants to drive through the country one comes up against the barrier
of the boundary fences which have gates with locks.

(Stephen Muecke in Benterrack *et al*. 1984: 66)

1   I leave home and walk through the streets of
Footscray. This is not the Foots Cray of London;
I don't know what relationship it has to that place.
With post-colonial bitterness I rebuke myself for
thinking of it, even as I progress through Clive,
Russell, Barclay, Shepherd, Gordon, Miller, and
White streets. I pass aged pensioners, Asian
grocers, a Greek cobbler, an Italian combined hair-
dressers and bottle-shop, the Beaurepaire tyre
factory, Edwardian and Victorian suburban houses,
the occasional brownbrick monument to a
European migrant's dreams, schoolchildren, drug
addicts and pushers, and a couple of major roads. I
see the business district close by, palm trees, jacar-
andas, rose bushes, sewerage workers giving notice
of deeper pathways, the remnants of a farm, and
about ten thousand cars. I arrive at my office. It has
taken me half an hour. I sit at my desk. Through
gum trees and European pines I can see Fleming-
ton racecourse and the Maribyrnong River. I write.

David drives from the country. He leaves his
small farm 80 km away and joins the Calder
Freeway into Melbourne from the west. It must
take him around an hour, although I have never
asked him. He crosses the plains, passes Kyneton;
sees 747s, the city towers, Bob Jane's Thunder-
dome, the estates of Sunbury, Taylors Lakes, Keilor
Downs, Kealba; he passes Organ Pipes National
Park, a fissure in the plains between Tullamarine
Airport and the freeway. Driving home in the
evenings the setting sun must get in his eyes. I have
wondered why this expatriate Englishman about to

return should choose to live so far away, and what
he thinks about on his trips up and down. How
does he cope with the great north winds in his
small car on summer days?

2   On the weekends before putting together the
final version of this edition of *Performance Research*
with David I drove around 2,000 km to areas north
and south of Melbourne.

First, over the Great Divide into the near
drought areas of Swan Hill, where small lot holders
and large wheat farmers plunder the Murray River
in a struggle to grow citrus fruit, grapes, and wheat
in an area which for millennia abundantly
supported Aboriginal people. The size and
openness of what are now largely bare plains
moving towards salinated infertility, and the sparse-
ness of the population around Swan Hill, are
probably unimaginable to urban Europeans;
Midwestern Americans might have a better chance.
And Swan Hill is by no means the 'outback' –
you'd have to travel another 1,000 km to get there.

Second, to Wilson's Promontory, a national park
at the southernmost tip of mainland Australia; a
place whose beauty, small huts and well-defined
tracks in defiance of the logic of the Australian
bush, have made it a refuge for white city-dwellers
for nearly a hundred years. The beauty of
Wilson's Promontory – a very fertile Greece with
sub-tropical rainforest and without the temples –
and the surrounding beaches and islands is the sort
of thing you see on tourist brochures.

Performance Research 3(2), pp.109-111 © Routledge 1998

Driving to these places you pass through acre after acre of European grasses and crops which have left Australian grasses to be found only in reserves and sometimes along the road verges where small corridors of native habitat allow animals to pass from coupe to coupe. I think of driving across the Nullabor with my mother in 1960: tracks in the sand, cattle grids and gates across the road, sand-dunes overtaking buildings at Eucla, an Aboriginal man at dusk standing on a bluff overlooking the road, spear and woomera in hand. Paxton reports that in the USA 'when Congress passed the Wilderness Act in 1964, it officially defined wilderness as any "roadless" area [5 miles from the nearest road] of at least 5,000 contiguous acres' (1986: 36 and 16).

3   Australia's ruling Conservative Party rushes headlong into privatization, the stripping of public assets, and the remorseless conversion of public places into private space. The state government of Victoria has embarked on a program of casino- and road-building in collusion with private companies that means I can drive from western Melbourne to the outer reaches of eastern Melbourne, perhaps 80 or 100 km, surrounded by constant roadwork, traffic, and concrete or steel barriers that prevent me seeing anything of the landscape behind them; all routes are marked by signs pointing me to the Casino, a tower of chance at the centre of the city. The racism, homophobia, and fear of difference being encouraged behind those barriers by our federal and state governments are real and effective weapons in the bid to distract attention from Australia's genocidal past (evidenced in the recent inquiry into the state-sponsored removal of Aboriginal children from their parents: Human Rights and Equal Opportunity Commission 1997), and its multinational present and future. The year 1998 could see a federal election in Australia based around the issue of race.

The freeway seems well made for such divisions:

Since so many of them are elevated, the driver on most urban expressways experiences a sensation of floating, of aerial rather than terrestrial movement, and a wide perspective that thrills the agoraphiliac heart. The freeway seems constructed for the purpose of offering a safe view of the city. It may also foster racial and ethnic segregation. The driver can look down into the slums like a visitor to one of those 'natural' zoos that run monorails among the lions and tigers.

(Paxton 1986: 109–10)

And yet, as Paxton acknowledges, driving through these constructions has its own pleasures. Merging, converging, bursting through, pressuring the driver in front of or beside me, controlling the flow of traffic by the gap between my vehicle and that in front, picking my way through the myriad possible routes, is an interactive movie as subtle as any contact improvisation; the apparent loss of volition in driving a seductive alternative to the clamor of postmodern, urban individualism:

Part of the freeway is about losing yourself in the crowd. People who could not stand to be on a bus or train full of strangers find merging their vehicle with the flow somehow refreshing, almost baptismal: a form of going down to the river.

(Paxton 1986: 111)

. . .

These thoughts from what is sometimes called the other side of the world. I leave you with an itinerary.

Standing in an open space face south-south east; take 15 steps, or walk until you strike a road, path, or corridor that runs east-west; turn east. Walk to the first crossroad, pathway, corridor, field, or building; cross over or through it, and continue straight ahead 280 steps or until the next crossroad, path, corridor, field, or barrier. Turn left, walk to the next bifurcation (crossroad, pathway, lane, corridor, or field) and turn so you can walk in a generally north-eastern direction veering into any street, alley, path, field, corridor, or doorway that you wish until close to 390 steps after you began walking north-east you meet a crossroad, path, or corridor; turn left. Ignore the first junction you come to, continue to the second; turn right. Walk to the end of this path or 710 steps; walk north-east for 180 paces or until you strike a path, turn right and walk to the end. At the first opportunity walk north-east again for approximately 40 paces, north-north-west for 60, north-east for 90, east-south-east for 50, and finally take 530 steps north-east. You have arrived. [You may need or want to adjust the particularities or scale of these instructions to your situation.]

Mark Minchinton, guest editor
Footscray, 24 March 1998

REFERENCES:

Benterrak, K., Muecke, S. and Roe, P., with Ray Keogh, Butcher Joe (Nangan), E. M. Lohe (1984) *Reading the Country: Introduction to Nomadology*, Fremantle: Fremantle Arts Centre Press.

de Certeau, M. (1984) *The Practice of Everyday Life*, Berkeley: University of California Press.

Human Rights and Equal Opportunity Commission (1997) *Bringing Them Home: A Guide to the Findings and Recommendations of the National Inquiry into the Separation of Aboriginal and Torres Strait Islander Children from their Families*, Sydney: HREOC.

Muecke, S. (1997) *No Road (Bitumen All the Way)*, Fremantle: Fremantle Arts Centre Press.

Paxton, P. (1986) *Open Road: A Celebration of the American Highway*, New York: Simon & Schuster.

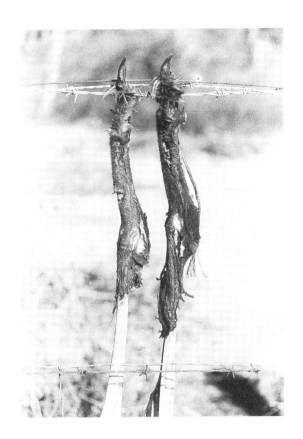

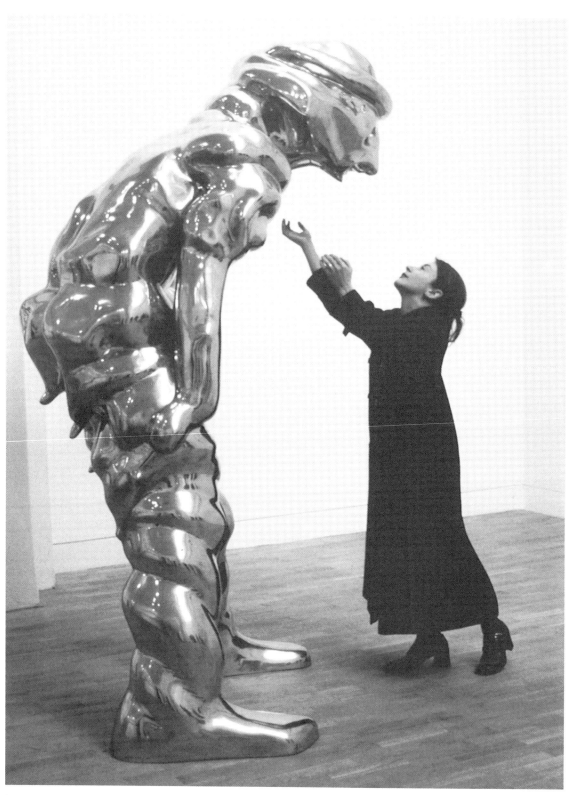

Scarlet Theatre. *Double Gazing*, performance for Thomas Schütte exhibition, Whitechapel Art Gallery, 1998. Photos: courtesy of Whitechapel Art Gallery.

Reviews

The Spectator as Performer

Nicholas Till

Double Gazing: a performance event by Scarlet Theatre, Thomas Schütte exhibition at the Whitechapel Art Gallery, London, January/February 1998

Anyone who visited the Duane Hanson show at the Saatchi Gallery in London last year will recognize the truth of Michael Fried's famous observation that minimalist art is inherently theatrical, transforming the spectator into a performer.

Duane Hanson a minimalist? The maker of hyperrealist replicas of the inhabitants of middle America, whose works are often dismissed as nothing more than Tussaud waxworks? Hanson's mannequins may be a long way from the minimalist objects of Donald Judd or Carl Andre. Yet Fried himself noted the way in which minimalism anthropomorphizes the sculptural object. The minimalist object deliberately eschews extremes of size, establishing instead a relationship to the scale of the human body and the space it occupies, to which Fried ascribed the effect of being 'crowded by the silent presence of another person', an effect that is obvious in Hanson's work (Fried 1967: 15). And just as the minimal object rejects dynamic composition in which the spectator's attention is engaged by the play of forces within the work, there is a similar rejection of dynamic energy or *contrapposto* in Hanson's blankly passive figures.

Fried recognized that the blankness of minimalist art throws back at the beholder an awareness of her own presence before the work. Although Hanson's figures are themselves ideally (in Fried's

terms) absorptive – whether through concentration on a task or through weary introspection – their uncanny realism repels the kind of absorptive attention that Fried demanded of significant art, recalling to the viewer that childhood injunction: 'Don't stare, it's rude.' At the Saatchi Gallery visitors preferred to view the figures from a distance, judging for themselves where they might situate a notional frame. Ultimately, as Fried anticipated, the gallery itself becomes the only relevant frame, presenting everything and everyone within it as a potential object of aesthetic scrutiny. The visitor who lingered in a state of immobility for any length of time soon attracted a small circle of amateurs marvelling at such verisimilitude. Visitors learned to play games with fellow visitors, teasing them with an illusion of inertness which uncannily inverted the illusion of life in Hanson's figures. Spectators indeed became performers.

The active role of the spectator in the construction of meaning is today a familiar subject of critical enquiry. But the mode of address of the minimal object repels the quest for closure in both meaning and aesthetic absorption, repositioning the spectator as a corporeal being within the real time and space of the gallery and thereby demanding not merely a cognitive or aesthetic, but also a performative, response. But what might be

Performance Research 3(2), pp.112–117 © Routledge 1998

the appropriate response for the spectator as performer before the artistic object which, besides refusing narrative, interpretive, or aesthetic closure, also declines to offer any clear spatial or temporal relationship to the viewer? Such, I believe, is the problem with which the work of the German artist Thomas Schütte presents us, and which Scarlet Theatre Company explored in a specially commissioned piece for performance within the Thomas Schütte exhibition at the Whitechapel.

Thomas Schütte's works employ a bewildering variety of media and forms. The visitor to the exhibition is confronted with objects which range from small wax mannequins, water-colour drawings, or photographs, to 8-foot aluminium figures and quasi-architectural models. But despite this variety the works share a number of features that serve to cast deliberate doubt on their ontological status. Several works have subject-matter that is presented in different media – e.g. three-dimensional and photographic – which leaves the viewer uncertain whether there is a definitive or final state for the work. Others have an unfinished quality which leaves us unclear whether they are projective sketches, or models, for works still to be made, whether they are unfinished works still to be completed, or whether their roughness is to be read as a significant property of the work itself. But the most striking feature of Schütte's work is his frequent manipulations of scale, which radically unsettle the spectator's ability to establish a perceptual or corporeal relationship to the objects being displayed.

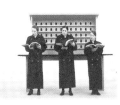

How do we read the scale of an object? Is a 3-foot construction, as Schütte himself asks, 'a miniature sculpture or a large-scale model' (Heyne *et al.* 1998: 22)? Is an 8-inch mannequin to be read as a reduced-scale model of a full-sized person or does it represent an imagined tiny person? A trio of such mannequins stands atop a massive chipboard plinth some 7 feet high; are they dwarfed by the size of the plinth, or rendered heroic? And how do we position

ourselves as viewers in relation to these different perceptions of the scale of a work?

In one of the first works in the show, entitled *Mohr's Life*, a mannequin painter stands at his easel surrounded by a series of tiny paintings: sombre skyscapes heavy with rain. The object of his paintings is a life-size rack of drying socks. As spectators we must choose whether to identify with the scale of Mohr's world, and if so, whether to ignore the fact that his tragic vision is founded upon the bathos of a horizon circumscribed by socks; or to identify with the more familiar scale of the rack of socks, and puzzle instead whether the fact that no sock matches any other has its referent in our world or that of Mohr.

In the next space nine 8-foot Mr Whippy anthropoids in gleamingly reflective aluminium seem to be engaged in some form of blurry interaction with each other; a dance or game, but the relationship is unclear. As spectators there is no ideal vantage point from which we can read the whole group and discern the artist's intentions. As the minimalist artist Robert Morris suggested, the distance between spectator and object in large-scale works means that 'physical participation becomes necessary' (Morris 1966: 21). But the effect of physical engagement is to disrupt our cognitive mastery of the object. In her study of the miniature and gigantic in art and literature Susan Stewart notes that the gigantic imposes a temporality upon our experience of objects, rendering our perception thereby partial and incomplete (Stewart 1993: 89). Moving amongst the group of *Grosse Geister* we are forced to conclude that the integrity of the figures as individual artworks is compromised by their evident relationship to each other, but we are given no vantage point from which to make sense of the whole group as one entity.

By contrast the miniature conventionally offers an illusion of mastery over both time and space. But in the main upstairs gallery at the Whitechapel a sequence of quasi-architectural models undermine that assumption. Three box-like objects stand at right-angles to each other, broadly the same in design, the inside edge of each containing five ledges with rows of openings. Their title, *For the Birds*, encourages us initially to view them at their own scale as dovecotes, functional objects stripped of unnecessary ornament. But they are clearly not merely functional; different and deliberate aesthetic choices have been made in the placement of colour, for instance. We can indeed admire them as aesthetic objects, Judd-like in their modular composition. But the insistent reminder of buildings such as Aldo Rossi's spooky Palazzo Hotel in Fukuoka, or the streetscapes of Mussolini's EUR, rebuff a purely aesthetic response, suggesting that we read the objects as models for edifices for human habitation. Together they form an empty arcaded piazza. Such buildings or ensembles are seen more often in photographic reproduction, which, like Schütte's models, turns them into innocuous stage sets, providing the viewer with a transcendent viewpoint which negates their oppressive monumentality. But if we refigure ourselves to the scale of the tiny humans who might inhabit Schütte's constructions we recognize that the piazza is as threatening as the paranoid cityscapes of de Chirico.

And here we are led to another disquieting aspect of Schütte's models. For even those which are manifestly closer to architecture, clearly resembling buildings designed for human use, retain a troubling blankness. Our first response may be to check the titles for clarification, but these are just as abstract: *W.A.S (Dwelling, Workshop, Studio); E.L.S.A. (Entrance, Life, Studio, Work)*. The verbal categories may be assumed to relate to the different spatial forms in the models, but the quest for further explanation is trapped within a vicious circle of referral. We may also note that the models are accompanied by drawings which supply specific details in their labelling ('storage' . . . 'street'), suggesting that they are not merely conceptual but that they relate to schemes for practical execution. But this renders the status of the models themselves uncertain, for as blueprints for construction they are not executed with the logic or consistency which would be required for such a purpose.

Susan Stewart suggests that just as narrative offers a sense of closure to our experience, abstraction supplies an illusion of transcendence. The effect of miniaturization should enhance that illusion, allowing the spectator to disengage from the field of representation (Stewart 1993: 13). But in Schütte's models there is a clear tension between abstraction and narrative that counteracts the possibility of disengagement. Michael Fried complained that the minimalist object is 'inexhaustible' not through fullness but because it allows of no closure (Fried 1967: 831), and this seems to be even truer of Schütte's works. If we read these models as conceptual structures we are encouraged to ignore their physical properties, seeking signifying explanation elsewhere. But frustrated in the search for conceptual closure the spectator is lured into a projective interaction with the work in search of narrative explanation. The very blankness of the exteriors of the buildings makes us bend to peer inside for clues. The act clearly replicates the impossible hermeneutic quest for inner meaning, but it also suspends our physical mastery over the object, luring us into self-miniaturization as we project ourselves into the space.

The models are, indeed, not hollow: stairs and ramps lead to doorways and vistas. But nothing is thereby explained; the interiors beg more questions than they answer.

Schütte's models make particular performative demands on the spectator. They are anxious objects that refuse any of the customary closures of aesthetic attention. Where much contemporary art deliberately transgresses aesthetic categories to open up new terrains for artistic enquiry Schütte's works refuse the liberation offered by such expanded fields. Superficially Schütte has much in common with other artists whose works straddle categories: Grenville Davey's not-furniture not-sculpture; Julian Opie's not-architecture not-sculpture. But in the work of people like Davey or Opie the object hovers between definable categories, and this element of categorical suspension allows the exemplary experience of Kantian aesthetics: the free play of the imagination as it is liberated from the categorical straitjacket of cognitive understanding. Schütte's works, however, are symptomatic of the shift from a structuralist to a poststructuralist articulation of meaning. In the former the not-term of difference holds the object of attention in place, providing it with boundaries which secure both likeness and difference, allowing the viewer to hold several references in play. The poststructuralist system is inherently unstable; the boundaries of likeness and difference no longer contain the object and closure bleeds away in endless deferral. Schütte's works are melancholy, neither attaining ontological plenitude nor offering the play of clear categorical reference.

The performative dilemma of the anxious spectator was explored with wit and imagination in *Double Gazing*. Three performers lead us through the exhibition in a developing sequence of possible responses to the work, enacting a search for appropriate modes of understanding or appreciation. Since the quest for closure is blocked at each stage, the viewers are forced to move on a somewhat Kantian journey from pure apperception to categorical understanding, from this to a search for aesthetic pleasure and imaginative freedom, and thence to the moral evaluation which Schütte himself ultimately seems to require of us.

The three performers are uniformly attired in black gabardines, which are obviously deemed appropriate wear for the serious task of art appreciation. They hug their exhibition catalogues to their chests like security blankets. On entering the space a cursory survey registers the bewildering range of the work. How do we decide where to begin looking in an exhibition which declines to offer a chronological point of origin or a curatorial statement of intention? For want of better guidance most of us embark in a clockwise direction, and a row of large black-and-white photographs high on the left-hand wall soon captures the attention of one of the performers. But she is immediately confronted with the familiar problem of how to view the images. Closeness places the viewer in an impossible, neck-craning position underneath the photos, forcing her to move back to find the

optimum vantage point. This sequence becomes a choreography of restless repositioning back and forth, until all three performers conclude that there *is* no ideal vantage point and turn their attention to the more obviously accessible objects in the space – the mannequins. In an attempt to gain a cognitive purchase upon these a process of patient identification begins: the figures are counted, their attributes are listed, the labels on their clothes are read out aloud, resemblances to the blown-up photographs are noted. But to enumerate empirical details of this kind is to seek understanding in the field of reference alone, ignoring the most obvious aspect of the figures: their miniaturization. The performers draw a blank.

Passing to the next space the performers encounter the *Grosse Geister*, Big Spirits. Here, rather than stimulating a cognitive response, the lack of definition in the figures, and their sheer size, encourage a more physical engagement. One of the figures seems to lean forward with a gesture of embrace, eliciting an attempted kiss which is thwarted by the figure's height; a second figure arouses imitative clapping, as if the performers were attempting to reconstruct the rules of the games in which the Spirits are absorbed. But as their names suggest, the actual size of the figures is contradicted by their apparent immateriality of form; their blurry and reflective lack of definition outwits the performers' attempts to sustain a satisfactory physical relationship.

(On the stairs leading to the upper gallery the constraints of aesthetic attention are temporarily suspended as the performers ask aloud the kinds of question that are reserved for such backstage areas: 'How much do you think this painting is worth?')

Upstairs the performers begin to abandon the quest for perceptual or cognitive understanding, or even direct physical engagement, and find themselves thereby liberated to explore more imaginative responses to the work. The emptiness of the bird-box piazza asks to be filled. But a purely physical response to the space would be too disruptive of its scale, so the piazza is filled instead with a delicate soundscape of dove-like coos, dispelling any lingering urban paranoia by restoring the boxes to the scale of domestic use. In the next pair of works, constructions of complex basement-like spaces inset into table tops, the performers are forced to acknowledge disjunctions between a physical and an imaginative response to the object. The sound turns to the pathetic mewing of a cat trapped somewhere in the basement whilst its searcher stands over the table and directs a torch into the space; basement, cat and searcher are, of course, physically incommensurate. Urban paranoia returns as the performers abandon any concern with scale, transforming the narrow space between two arcaded box-like objects into the dangerous terrain of an armed police raid.

But how much latitude do Schütte's works really offer for such initiatives? We might well consider that these games, far from being truly imaginative, are indicative instead of the literal-minded response of those who demand a simple narrative key to everything, ignoring the properties of the objects themselves or the possibility of concealed meanings susceptible only to more sustained attention. The model for an artist's studio entitled *E.L.S.A.* does indeed seem to recall the performers to their duties as responsible spectators. Enacting the hermeneutic quest for explanation within, one of the performers directs a series of questions into the interior of the building, assumed to be the refuge of the artist himself: 'Are you the artist . . . you know that letter – did you write it ? . . . What's the significance of the socks? . . .' But the artist, of course, is not at home. Responsibility for meaning rests with the spectator.

In classical aesthetics the spectator is constructed as an ahistorical and genderless abstraction. But Scarlet's three female performers now remind us that a female response to an art object may differ from a male response. The model entitled *W.A.S* represents an ideal living and working compound which raises questions about the artist's implied relationship to the domestic sphere. Does the presence of a domestic space alongside the artist's workspace not suggest, perhaps, that the function of the domestic sphere is to service the needs of the working artist? Our female spectators sniff a male

plot, ventriloquizing the wife who must surely be cast to combine the roles of servant, mistress, mother and muse within this ideal establishment.

In its drab appearance an adjacent construction entitled *Landhaus IV* is unexceptional, except for the gleaming toy Porsche, parked outside, an actual replica whose appearance brings an incongruous element of realism to the ensemble, until we realize that it is no more or less 'real' than any of the other models we have looked at. The car's provocative presence elicits an ironical response at the expense of sexualized male toys as the performers transform themselves into car-show hostesses, leaving us to decide if they are laughing at or with the artist.

We have reached the end of the exhibition. What have we seen? What do we feel? What do we think? This pressure to articulate a coherent response inhibits most spectators. The public formality of the gallery space itself, and the need to protect objects of aesthetic and financial value, deter physical encounters which might be less intimidating. The gallery walls are liberally posted with reminders not to touch the objects, and the attendants exercise admonitory vigilance. The performers shuffle out of the gallery chanting a liturgy of gallery prohibitions: 'No smoking . . . no photography . . . no leaning . . . no asking questions . . . no playing . . . no making up stories on the spot . . . no crying . . .' But are these the prohibitions of the gallery, or are they in fact a response to the refusals of Schütte's works? Our vicarious double-gazing has surely demonstrated that, far from denying freedom, Schütte's aesthetic and conceptual prohibitions may serve to stimulate feats of virtuoso spectatorship.

REFERENCES

Fried, Michael (1967) 'Art and objecthood', *Artforum* 5(10).
Heyne, Julian, Lingwood, James and Vettese, Angela (1998) *Thomas Schütte*, London: Phaidon Press.
Morris, Robert (1966) 'Notes on sculpture 2', *Artforum* 5(2).
Stewart, Susan (1993) *On Longing: Narratives of the Miniature, the Gigantic, the Souvenir, the Collection*, Durham, NC and London: Duke University Press.

The *Informe* Body

Tracey Warr

Formless: A User's Guide
Yve-Alain Bois & Rosalind E. Krauss, eds.
New York: MIT Press, Zone Books 1997
£22.50 (hbk) 304 pp. ISBN 0942299434

Cindy Sherman Retrospective
Essays by Amanda Cruz, Elizabeth A. T. Smith and
Amelia Jones
New York & London: Thames & Hudson 1997
£22.50 (pbk) 219 pp. ISBN 050027987X

Body Art: Performing the Subject
Amelia Jones
Minneapolis & London: University of Minnesota
Press 1998
£17.20 (pbk) 349 pp. ISBN 0816627738

**Out of Actions: Between Performance and
the Object 1949–1979**
Paul Schimmel ed.
Los Angeles/London: Los Angeles Museum of Contemporary Art/Thames & Hudson 1998
£29.95 (pbk) 368pp. ISBN 0500280509

The 90s has been a rich decade for revisionist interpre-
tations of body art with the Pompidou's *Hors Limites*
(1994); *Inside the Visible* (1996); the Guggenheim's *Rrose
is a Rrose is a Rrose* (1997) and important critical essays
by writers including Kristine Stiles and Amelia Jones.
Theoretical examinations of the artist's indexical trace
have also informed our consideration of body art. Two
new major contributions are the recent Los Angeles
Museum of Contemporary Art's survey show and
catalogue *Out of Actions: Between Performance and the
Object 1949–79* and Jones' new book, *Body Art: Performing the Subject*.

Contemporaneous critics of body art were often
hostile, baffled or, at best, reserved. How did it relate to
the discourse of aesthetics? Or did it, in fact, relate more
closely to a discourse of psychology and anthropology?
Even sympathetic critics came to the conclusion that
artists' use of themselves as art objects was the equivalent
of self-abuse and verging on the neurotic. Feminist com-
mentators criticised women body artists who used their
own nude bodies in their work and seemed to collude
with the objectification of women.

60s and 70s art practice and art theory were pulling in
different directions. Artists were dematerializing art and
confronting an objective, academic aesthetic with the
libidinous, contingent, subjective impact of their bodies,
whilst formalist critics continued to strive to keep art
defined as autonomous, universal, finite, object.

Body art has been gradually eroding the idea of self or
body as stable, finite, essentialist forms. It addressed temporality, contingency, instability, flux, non-closure, performativity. It explored the notion that identity is acted
out and performed in time. It explored that element of
the self and the body – consciousness – that is invisible,
formless, continuous, liminal. The self-doubt of art –
what is art? – arising from artists' attacks on conventions,
coincides with the doubt of self – who and what am I?

Georges Bataille argued that the origin of art is the
indexical, externalizing sign – the hand dipped in the
paint pot and imprinted on a cave or nursery wall, mate-
rializing the existence of the self. Yves Klein enacted this
with the shirt he made in 1948 with the paint prints of
his hands and feet. 'Leave my mark on the world, I have
done it! . . . When I was a child . . . Hands and feet thick
with colour, applied to the surface, suddenly there I was,
face to face with my own psyche.'

Writing about Robert Rauschenberg, Helen
Molesworth contends that 'The origin of the work of art
is the artist's body – in the pressing and smearing, in the
dailiness of bodily functions, in the question "What kinds
of marks can I make?"' (Molesworth 1993). She argues
that Rauschenberg 'attempted to turn himself inside out
to mark his own body on the canvas'. In the work of
Jackson Pollock, Rauschenberg, Kazuo Shiraga and

Performance Research 3(2), pp.118-121 © Routledge 1998

Francis Bacon, the viscosity of paint apes the viscerality of the body, its liquid, glutinous, congealing mess referring to bodily fluids. Bacon wrote 'I would like my pictures to look as if a human being had passed between them, like a snail, leaving a trail of the human presence and memory trace of past events, as the snail leaves its slime'. Marcel Duchamp's *Sinning Landscape* (1946) made with semen on black velvet prefigures the preoccupation with leaking bodies of more recent artists. As Ben Vautier commented, 'Art is dirty work but somebody has to do it'.

As art object the artist's body is, of course, always ephemeral. Alan Sonfist has bequeathed his body to the Museum of Modern Art in his will, Orlan is planning to leave her mummified body to a museum and Bob Flanagan left instructions for art projects after his death involving the display of his decomposing body. But until delivery of a corpse is taken the artist's body will always get up and walk away back into life, leaving only its imprint or trace in paint, gelatin, microchips, its relic in cast objects, its indexical mark or stain, or simply its memory burnt on the retina and the cortex.

Some critics have argued that real witnessed performance is the cathartic and authoritative experience, as opposed to the secondary, vicarious experience of documentation. But many artists' body works were witnessed by very small audiences or by none at all – they were staged for the camera and the video recorder. So what is the status of these photographs, documents, films, video and relics of artists' actions? *Out of Actions* is an important contribution to this debate.

The artist's body is a conscious material object, self-evidently self-reflexive and in dialogue with its audience. Whether the audience is sharing the same physical space with the artist's body in real time, or whether they are contemplating it in documentation or other relic, that audience is unable to have a purely objective response to the artist's body. Each viewer must project knowledge of their own body into that other body they are looking at. In live performance one is distracted in this projection by the fact that you have an audience yourself. You have to maintain your *sang froid* and are caught in the act of voyeurism, at the peephole of Duchamp's *Etant Donnés*, the bumhole of Paul McCarthy's *Rear View* through which one bends over to peer at a tiny Swiss village inside, or sitting in the audience of a disturbing performance by Ron Athey or Franko B. Whilst the vicarious experience of the documentation audience is one of direct, private, undisturbed empathy with the imagined experience.

In her new book, Jones discusses the performativity of both male and female gender, focusing on a small selection of artists including Carolee Schneemann, Yayoi Kusama, Acconci, Hannah Wilke, James Luna, Lyle Ashton Harris and Flanagan and Sheree Rose. Like her earlier book on Duchamp, Jones's *Body Art* benefits from this detailed discussion of individual artist's work. Jones's discussion is an important clarification of the double standard of body art interpretation where the norm for both artist and spectator was assumed to be male gendered, and where male body art was read as depersonalized, universal and transparent whilst women's body art was perceived as masochistic, obscene, exhibitionist, narcissistic and anti-feminist.

Many 70s artists such as Judy Chicago engaged in an essentialist celebration of the female body. But gender as biologically innate began to be questioned. Judith Butler argues that gender identity is performative rather than substantive, that it is a theatrical construct sustained by repetitive demonstration. This thesis is explored in the tradition of gender disruption and performativity in photography and film documented in the Guggenheim's *Rrose is a Rrose is a Rrose* (Blessing 1997).

Body art has been largely considered within the discourse of identity politics and ideologies inscribed and resisted in bodies and selves, which has obscured the extent to which artists are often using their bodies and their selves in terms of their consciousness rather than their identities, to explore the conditions that are shared by all bodies of any gender, race, sexuality or class – birth, transient and visceral life, intense consciousness and death.

Artists use their bodies both to critique identity construction and to explore the body as a real, mortal thing. Mary Kelly argued that artists who invoke 'the phenomenological body' were engaging in a form of essentialist romanticism. But to only see the body as a construct has to be questioned. Artists such as Burden, Pane, Marina Abramovic, Raul Zurita and Diamela Eltit reject the postmodernist thesis that there is nothing but simulacra and power. They insert the body's vulnerability, mortality, mutability, isolation as a humanistic agenda. Body art flouts our notion of the individual as the cumulative centre of everything and our idea of the unassailable integrity of the body. As Orlan remarks we think the sky will fall on our heads if we mess with the body.

Elaine Scarry has described pain as the deconstructor of consciousness, stripping the body of its self-reassuring constructs, objects, world and leaving it exposed for what it is – vulnerable, mortal, mutable, alone. Burden's works, *Gateway to Heaven*, *Shoot*, *Velvet Water*, for example, 'take art to the verge of suicide' exposing the fact of human mortality. The fact that he is stating the obvious does not lessen its impact or make it pointless to say it.

Mortality is not a construct, a projection or a fantasy, although some religious belief systems would have it so. Mortality is an unavoidable fact, common to us all. As Denis Hollier puts it, 'If you die, you die, you can't have a substitute'. The artist's body does explore and perform identity, it does explore ideology inscribed on and in the body – but it also performs mortality in the trace, the absence, the erasure, the memory of the embodied consciousness.

Ana Mendieta's work, marking various natural landscapes with the schematic, iconographic traces of her own body, was essentialist in intention and reception. Her work emphasizes the absence and erasure of her body and her self, their loss in temporality and mortality. Materiality has escaped and the relics and residue of actions remain as reminders. In this case a double erasure occurs as the body imprints were generally ephemeral and only preserved in photographic and film documentation. Mendieta's work emphasizes a transformation from event to memory.

Lucy Lippard and John Chandler's 1968 essay 'The Dematerialization of Art' described body art, along with land art and concept art, as for a while at least a strategy for eluding the art market and establishment's need to consume, fetishize and exploit objects. In focusing on the art market and objecthood, however, critics missed an important point that artists were not merely dematerializing the valuable art object but addressing the immaterial and the nature of materialization itself. The 'dematerialization of art' has now come an interesting full circle. The art market quickly adapted to apportion value to relics and documentation. Orlan sells ounces of her excised flesh in reliquaries, Jeff Koons manipulates art consumers, artists' film and video sell at inflated prices.

Beyond the dematerialization of art, body art's challenge to the notion of form is not widely acknowledged and, perhaps surprisingly, not addressed in Yve-Alain Bois and Rosalind Krauss's *Formless: A User's Guide*. Bois and Krauss build on Bataille's concept of the informe to develop a thesis of the formless in 20th century artworks which is a major contribution to contemporary art debate.

Bois and Krauss's book mimics the volatile taxonomy and categorical ruptures of Bataille's own non-dictionary published in *Documents*. They describe how the indeterminate lumps and blobs of art works from Fontana's *Ceramica Spaziale* (1949) to Mike Kelley's *Riddle of the Sphinx* (1971) are subversive of form. They discuss a tradition of 20th century art practice which is voiding the anthropomorphic and narrative and located on the boundary where figure and ground are blurring in entropy. They explore the contiguity of object and context, the boundary between animate and inanimate and the role of the artist's indexical trace in the art object in terms of absence and mortality. They delineate the informe not as nihilistically meaningless but as a perpetual maintenance of potentials. Whilst Bois concentrates on a Bataillean perspective, Krauss ranges through readings also employing structural linguists and psychoanalysis. Bois rushes us along a line and Krauss digs deep in one place.

With the exceptions of Lygia Clark and Cindy Sherman's work they do not discuss artists body work. In a discussion on the informe and the abject in *October* magazine, Krauss admitted that the body is her phobic object (Krauss et al. 1994). Artists use their own bodies in art as an ambiguous form – a form on its way to formlessness – death, and coming out of formlessness – birth, with a foot – one the material body the other the immaterial consciousness – in both camps of dedifferentiated and defined and boundaried matter. The body and consciousness are precarious form always on the brink of dissolution and in connection with their own link to the informe. If a contemplation of death is projected into art discourse, into art objects, the personal nature of death can remain repressed, euphemistic, evaded, as it cannot be if this contemplation is projected instead onto the body.

Krauss argues that the abject is about the impassibility of the body's frontiers, offering a deluded freedom of evacuation. But the body's frontiers are passable. The body is a permeable membrane, a fluid consciousness. Jean-Paul Sartre pointed out that the autonomous subject is compromised by slimy substances and Julia Kristeva had equated the abject and bodily disgust of the slimy and unformed with the mother – the threat to autonomous form. Barbara Creed's essay on the 'monstrous feminine' explores this threat in the maternal, birth imagery of the *Alien* horror films (Creed, 1986).

We fear dissolution and incoherence, the proximity of the inanimate and the animate, the human and the thing, the live and the dead. Themes of disfiguration, dissolution, degeneration and the flimsiness of the border between animate and inanimate in Surrealism are impressed directly on the body in the work of later 'messy' body artists such as Otto Muhl, McCarthy, Schneemann or recently Sherman. The dualistic notion of subject/object is gradually broken down and replaced by the idea of a reciprocating loop, with the body as leaking membrane between the two nodes.

When an artist walks into their studio they bring with them all their perceptions, experiences, memories, rationalizations, knowledge, but they bring also their body twitching with electrical and chemical reactions, crawling with an invisible quantum life and motivation, the microflora and fauna of genes, cells, DNA and enzymes.

In contemporary art the body is often at the juncture of a radical interface with technology and an exploration of the nature of consciousness. The body is diversely altered, extended, dwarfed, threatened, secularized, colonized by science and technology. Rather than revealing that we are frightened by our own technology, theories that reduce us to machinery show instead a fear of our own bodies' mortality and generative power. The technological project is the old project of evading the conditions of the human body – birth and death.

In Barney's work the body is subject to a medical aesthetic of bloodless gore and prosthetic colours. Objects are wounded, seeping and excreting gelatinous matter – wax, lubricants, petroleum jelly. Barney explores the body's tendency to excess, surfeit and waste. The body appears as a hybridized, consuming, excreting, conceiving, transforming conduit for matter.

Orlan's work pulls back the hospital curtain and intrudes into the privacy of expert medical intervention in the body which usually excludes spectators and patient alike from the spectacle of the opened body. Her body is sculpted in cosmetic surgery under local anaesthetic producing 'an image of a cadaver under autopsy which keeps on speaking'.

The embodied consciousness is an enormously temporary and precarious cohesion. The material body – along with all matter – is in a constant state of mutability and is ruthlessly confronted with its own impending caesura. We expect the visible to be solid and real but only the patterns of matter are stable–the material is not. Manuel DeLanda starkly describes us as 'temporary coagulations of recycling matter . . . The flow of flesh through food chains constitutes the main form of energy circulation in organic strata' (DeLanda 1992). As anthropologist Mary Douglas pointed out, we are surrounded by and swimming in the detritus of millions of dead, disappeared people.

Many artists in the 90s present to us their visceral leaking bodies. Paul McCarthy's work depicts 'a body whose borders were collapsing, whose insides seemed to be gushing out as though its thin bag of skin had ruptured' (Rugoff 1996: 32–87). Sherman's recent work powerfully explores this theme. There are several books on parts of Sherman's oeuvre, but *Cindy Sherman Retrospective* brings all her work together, accompanied by her working notes, which allows us to see the extraordinary development from a consideration of the forms of female self and representation to a consideration of the nonboundary between inner and outer, between form and formless, between human and thing.

Liquid is indivisible and not structured like language, body and form. The significance of gravity and liquidity in the work of Pollock, Ed Ruscha, Robert Morris, Andy Warhol, Eva Hesse, Klein and Sherman is discussed by Bois and Krauss. But they do not refer to the perception of the body as liquid, as flow of flesh and consciousness, presented in the work of some body artists. In the viscerality of much contemporary body art the temporal, fluid values of consciousness are pitted against the stasis of commodity or object fetishism.

REFERENCES

Blessing, Jennifer, ed. (1997) *Rrose is a Rrose is a Rrose: Gender Performance in Photography*, New York: Guggenheim.

Creed, Barbara (1986) 'Monstrous Birth', *Screen*, Jan–Feb, pp. 44–70.

DeLanda, Manuel (1992) 'Nonorganic Life' in Jonathan Crary and Sanford Kwinter, eds., *Incorporation*, New York: Zone, pp. 129–167.

Krauss, Rosalind, Foster, Hal, Molesworth, Helen, Hollier, Dennis (1994) 'The Politics of the Signifier II: A Conversation on the Informe and the Abject', *October*, 67 (Winter), Cambridge, MA: MIT Press, pp.3–21.

Molesworth, Helen (1993) 'Before Bed', *October* 63 (Winter), Cambridge, MA: MIT Press, pp. 69–82.

Rugoff, Ralph (1996) 'Mr McCarthy's Neighborhood' in *Paul McCarthy*, London: Phaidon, pp. 32–87.

Book Review

Unmaking Mimesis: Essays on Feminism and Theatre

Elin Diamond
London and New York:
Routledge, 1997

226 pp. ISBN: 0-415-01229-5 (pb); 0-415-01228-7 (hb)

At the beginning of this book Elin Diamond disarms her readers with an epigraph from Nietzsche: 'What in us really wants the truth?' 'Not me,' replies the dissembling reader, since for those who aspire to perform or write about performance in a postmodern world, 'truth' is not what is sought. Truth is the smokescreen confusing those who want to see the world on stage as 'true' to life, or the actor as revealing a personal 'truth', or the display of emotion as 'true' to character, or the content of the play as a 'truth' about society. According to Diamond, we must undo or unmake the illusion of truth in the theatre if we are to understand the truth-tellings of its mimesis. These essays offer a collection of theoretical strategies (deconstruction, feminist theory, materialist criticism) as well as tools embedded in the very processes and structures of theatrical communication (realism, performance theory, acting styles, dramatic genre, dramatic language) to approach this question of mimesis.

She begins by returning to the ancient philosophical conundrum of mimetic resemblance as either false illusion or universal truth revealed in art. Utilizing the commentaries of Derrida and Irigaray, Diamond interprets mimesis as both a mode of representation and an activity for producing truths from a representation. But feminist theory has made us sceptical of the equation of mimesis with the feminine (who is excluded from representing herself except by mimicry) and Brechtian theory alerts us to the historical and social conditions hidden in representation. Thus Diamond argues that a critical mimesis will be a double process: able to 'unravel image, identity and subject' as well as to reveal, test and excite certain 'truths' about the performer's gendered body and the situating of lived experience in performance.

Throughout the book, these double operations of mimesis inform Diamond's 'ethical accounting' of the historical materials and desires of representational practice. In the first chapter, she examines several key melodramas and early realist plays and their representation of the 'fallen woman' to illustrate the ways in which realism, as a dominant theatrical mode, has translated the body of the hysterical woman into acceptable bourgeois form. But, she argues, theatrical realism has also dropped the wall on the disturbing 'secret' of the female hysteric: nowhere is this more visible than in the double representation of Hedda Gabler, whose secret is both a pregnant sexuality and her use of a weapon, the pistol, as symbolic agent of the phallus. As Susan Melrose suggests, female actors or characters can wield the phallus, if only temporarily. Diamond does not reject realism, as some feminists have, but instead suggests that it encodes the verbal and gestural signs of the hysteric which reveal the 'unspeakable' of the female body that bourgeois society would repress. 'The signs of guilt are the signs of the body' (25) is a declaration that begs further consideration.

Diamond was significantly one of the first feminist theatre scholars to reappropriate Brecht's techniques – the *Verfremdungseffekt*; the 'not but'; historicization and gestus – for reading the corporeal signs of sexual difference in terms which exceed the political dialectics of dramatic structure. In her gestic feminist criticism, the actor-character is no longer the tablet of the author's inscription nor the fetishized recipient of the spectator's gaze but instead the performer connotes a 'looking-at-being-looked-at-ness' which is 'paradoxically available for both analysis and identification' (52). This double looking in the act of signification enables the reader or spectator to historicize the production of images of gender within dramatic texts as well as to consider the strategies employed by women dramatists and actors to retain their own doubleness as female subjects within theatre and culture.

Diamond exemplifies this 'mode of reading' in essays on Aphra Behn, the historical 'mother' of female dramatists, and Caryl Churchill, the leading contemporary British feminist playwright. In these essays, mimesis (veils, masks, allegory, disguise, artifice) and bodies (dressed, undressed, painted, disguised, orificial, bursting, fantastic) dance through the historical constraints of potentially deadening patriarchal frames of representation. This is followed by a lengthy discussion of Adrienne Kennedy's theatre work, a mimesis which dismantles not only dramatic structure but also questions of racial identification from the position of a 'black Atlantic' subject. Whilst I was theatrically inspired by the material on Churchill at an earlier time, particularly Diamond's teasing out of the 'invisible bodies' in *A Mouthful of Birds*, these chapters require some preliminary knowledge of these authors and their works in order to fully engage with the discussion. Without knowing Kennedy's plays, it was difficult to determine in what ways Diamond was miming the source material in her corporeal criticism or whether she was exposing sufficiently the historical conditions of African-American theatrical identities. When one of the characters in Kennedy's *Funnyhouse of a Negro* says 'I want not to be', Diamond admits to being faced with a theatre which confounds European assertions of a rational selfhood traditionally embodied in the presence of the speaking subject. Given such an incommensurability of starting positions interpellated by racial differences (writer as speaker, writer as actor, writer to critic, actor to spectator, critic for reader), it seems that more specific description would enhance the details of analysis in this chapter.

Her final chapter on 'performance and temporality' inverts the previous chapters with their focus on

playwrights and textual bodies to deal directly with new models of performance produced in the historical and cultural bodies of three feminist performance artists: Robbie McCauley, Deb Margolin, Peggy Shaw. Diamond acknowledges the popular temptation to celebrate the fractured intertextuality of identity in contemporary theory and art, and so gives us a history lesson in American culture (and its love of the car) with a critical assessment of postmodern performance style. Having put on trial the *longue durée* of philosophical discourse on representation with its focus on the visual signs of the actor's presence within the spatial frame, Diamond now undertakes the deconstruction of theatrical time. In postmodern performance, duration is no longer regulated by three acts or one act, or even by the unfolding of episodic or epic time. Instead, according to Diamond, the performance artist exposes the historicity of the performative action in the present moment: these performers address the discursive operations which have produced (past tense) their subjectivity as a mode of speaking but also insist upon the immediacy of a future present in which female acts of mimesis no longer reflect a selfsame subject. Time is therefore critically active when a Somebody is watching an Other body with all the activation of 'systems of sensing, recognising, and knowing about the self and the Other' that makes performance a mode of desiring.

True or false, as Marie Maclean once claimed, is not the dialectic of performance but the potential success or failure of the effects of desire and its lack in the communication. So what are we looking for in performance? I have a sense of

millennial finality in reading *Unmaking Mimesis* which shifts so easily from theatre to performance studies, from modernism to the edge of postmodernism, from the critical spectator to the cathartic 'truths' of mimesis, after which there seems no more 'reason' to justify performance. In this, I am, of course, mistaken, for it is in the power to represent and present that performance can insist on a partial and very important form of truth by showing us 'what happens when?' If this is another answer to the problem of mimesis, then Diamond's call for a performance of 'subjects-in-relation' might be just what is needed in the twenty-first century as more shadows (male, female, black, white, colonized, colonizer) are unleashed from their mimetic chains in the 'apparently impossible simultaneity' of human historical differences.

Rachel Fensham

Archive Review

THE ARCHIVE AS EVENT

The Black Kit/Die Schwarze Lade
ASA-European
Art Service Association, Köln

'A maximum of mental sources and information in exchange with a minimum of materialisation. A basic sense of new definition in performance art and the first step in preparing a network as a physical and mental form.' So starts the information on 'The Black Kit' – an archive of ASA and its (former) parallel association Black Market International. Elsewhere in the literature and documentation that surrounds the (net)work of ASA-European – the Art Service Association centred on Köln, inspired and given direction by performance artist Boris Nieslony – it states that ASA 'is not an art project'. Instead, it 'puts values into transfer' and in this way 'communication has a precise effect on all cultural activities, including art'. The place of a material archive in such a fluid and conceptual network is summarized by a further statement:

> ASA is a communications pool into which energy, materials and information are constantly being fed. It is impossible to receive anything directly from this pool, to draw anything out or to expect anything from it. Nonlinearly and non determinable by ASA, free floating forms materialise in unexpected places, for which ASA now sets the required framework. Within these boundaries free floating forms take shape. They consist of information, ideas and matter and they solidify into wares, projects or events and form meaningful relationships. Thereafter, these materializations disappear once more into the pool, 'ASA'. (ASA 1997)

The image of a fluid 'communications' pool, which aptly characterizes the work that Boris Nieslony tirelessly continues to initiate, remains in some senses utopian. Such fluidity coagulates, gradually forming into the weights and measures of history – the archive becomes a material point of focus, of memory – and in this case literally becomes a growing but still movable 'kit' (see photo) where information and resources on a wide range of performance artists can become organized and catalogued. The material fact of the archive now becomes a focus for the 'development of a centre for studies, education and information' – always a precarious balance between the openness of arts action and fixities of the academy.

> 'Only art gives us the possibility to say something that we don't know' claimed the satirist Gabriel Laub. We also work with art as a medium of expression. But, since we have a particular tool at our disposal, we can say without being insolent: 'Art gives us the possibility to say something that we know'. And as this knowledge in its peculiarity compounds of several charitable components, we like to make this knowledge available to (for) anybody interested. The Black Kit is primarily an important tool for educational work, research and documentation focussing on performance

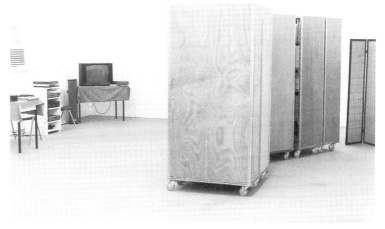

The Black Box. Photo: B. Nieslony

Performance Research 3(2), pp.124-126 © Routledge 1998

art, project art and artist-run spaces. (ASA 1997)

The idea for The Black Kit originated in 1981 at a project in Stuttgart for seventy invited artists working in performance, performance art, installation, painting and video, called The Council (Das Konzil). The project, initiated by Boris Nieslony , sought to extend and develop areas of interactive communication. The participants did not wish to catalogue the proceedings of The Council but proposed instead a transportable container which could be taken from event to event, from meeting to meeting. The Black Kit was envisaged as a generator of thoughts, as an archive and as a sculpture of public interest.

Exhibition spaces are turned into a public library offering to anyone the power of the ideas documented here. Not just an invitation for the viewer to consume, but an invitation for thoughtful studies of letters, photos, poems, videotapes, objects, relics and records of open work-situations. Moreover it includes the opportunity for debate about the topics and offerings experienced. (Jürgen Raap, *Kunstforum* 95, 1988)

The Black Kit has been presented several times within the framework of exhibitions from 1988 onwards. This means of presenting the 'archive as event' not only signifies the literal display of selected parts of the stock but also the active and interactive realization of certain areas of the archive and their implications.

The Black Kit contains documentation since 1975 of the most important international projects with communicative structures related to performance. There are documentations of artists' self-help organiz-

ations, artist-run spaces, conferences, seminars and interactive projects. Since 1981 the archive has collected and structured documents of both realized and unrealized projects. The archive has become an organism, a permanently growing account of ideas. Including documentation in a wide range of media, the archive is structured with an index that provides the possibility of searching through thematic and conceptual links and connections, keywords, fields/ domains, and networks. At present The Black Kit includes documentation, dates and information on more than one thousand artists; over one hundred video-documents of performance events in Europe, Asia, and North America; plus numerous slides, records and audiotapes; more than five hundred journals/ magazines, periodicals, catalogues and brochures concerned with the practice and theory of performance art. The archive catalogue is also available on-line.

ASA-European publishes an annual performance reader *Slaps – Banks – Plots* . At present there are two readers based on ASA-initiated performance conferences (1997 and 1998) which contain a wide range of contemporary writings and statements by artists. The readers are available on disc direct from ASA (for DM 20,-) and also on-line. The ASA website itself has many interesting links to ASA's network activities and to other performance related archives. The CH [Swiss] Performance Netzwerk will host The Black Kit with Boris Nieslony at Pfäffikon on 28–29 February 1999.

Ric Allsopp

INFORMATION:
ASA-European e.V.
Rathenauplatz 35

D-50674 Köln
email: asabank@dom.de
tel. 0049 (0) 221 245115
fax: 0049 (0) 221 240 4422
The most immediate means of accessing events, information and projects that comprise the ASA networks is via the World Wide Web:
http://www.asa.de
Further information concerning ASA-European and The Black Kit archive is available via:
http://www.asa.de/ASA/ index.htm
Information on recent and forthcoming events and projects is available via:
http://www.asa.de/ASA/ NewsFrame.htm

THE EVENT AS ARCHIVE

Performance Index
Basel, Switzerland

In the near distance the rumble of demolition vehicles resumes after the noon break. Two entire blocks of an already outdated 1950s convention centre are being chomped down and trucked away. The vanishing complex dates roughly from the same time as what some say is the beginning of performance art history, i.e. Jackson Pollock, John Cage, Allan Kaprow. The history of performance art in Basel (to date, unwritten) begins later with Tinguely, Rot, Spoerry, de Sinphal et al., who performed in the 1970s in this city, which for its size gives considerable support to the arts including provisions for small-scale projects, loosely organized and tended slowly, simmering on a low back-burner.

One such 'simmerer' is Performance Index , a name constituted by a group of friends who had the idea of organizing a festival and who gathered round a table set up by performance artist Heinrich Lüber at the end of 1994. The name is borrowed from Swiss Performance Index, the Swiss equivalent of the US Dow Jones or the German DAX and, like the stock market measure, the intention is to give a pointer as to how performance art is doing.

In September 1995 Performance Index presented a festival of forty events packed into four dense days [see http://www.thing.at/performance-index]. The events ranged across a broad spectrum of performance subgenres from ritual to pseudo-scientific lecture; from the 'visual poetics of objects and actions' to audience terrorization; from body mutilation to tacky and camp.[1] As the festival was constructed with an eye towards bridging a gap between two generations, tried and seasoned works could be seen alongside untried and evolving pieces. This variety-pack atmosphere was underscored by the venue: most events took place in the Warteck, a large, nineteenth-century, former brewery in a state of messy renovation, whose spaces of various size and character were once sites for the beer-making process. Today the Warteck is an almost fancy alternative arts centre.

In the making of the 1995 festival, Performance Index published the beginnings of its archive – an assemblage of pages held together in an open ring-binder. The pages included some essays by experts interleaved with two-sided descriptions and photos of performance artists written and submitted by the artists themselves. The idea of this fluid archive is that new pages can always be added or old ones updated. Presently the book (available from Performance Index for SF 45,-) includes pages on about one hundred contemporary European performance artists. In addition, the Performance Index website provides useful information on the artists who comprise the archive, and on related performance projects and events and links. Performance Index invites artists and theorists to take part in an international exchange and to send in their own contributions. The objective is to stage a topical discussion on Performance Art through the intermediary of the forum (as 'book' as website, as event).

In late March 1999, in association with a series of events (CH Performance Netzwerk),[2] Performance Index will present a second festival. The programming group includes ten persons, and discussion about a concept is under way. The primary venue, in the heart of the old inner city, will be the upper empty floors of the Architecture Museum and architecture bookstore and publisher Domus-Haus, a former commercial building designed by Rasser + Vadi (1959) and under protection as a significant modernist work. The Architecture Museum is a transparent, crystal building with a reinforced concrete skeleton. Thin iron and concrete pillars bear the floor-slabs from which the all-glass facade is hung. Because the support-and-bearing construction is independent from the wall, the floor plan of the entire building is open and flexible. There's no strategy as yet to develop a concept in immediate response to the venue, described in the museum brochure as a 'Manifestation of the Modern'; 'Now we can afford to have one point of view, we don't have to do a survey again', says Heinrich Lüber. However, with ten persons round the programming table, this one point of view promises to be multivalent, polyphonic.

Coming back to the general idea of Performance Index, it will be interesting in 1999 to have a new measure of how performance art is doing; a cross-section, a pulse taken in these times of increasingly rapid change. Since the 1995 festival performance art has become a more defined project, discourse and discipline in Switzerland: it is being taken more seriously. As a genre, it is in the running for inclusion in museum programs and now it has a place as a category in competitions and awards. If a few million square feet of architecture like the convention centre can be taken down and replaced in ten months because its structure – only twenty-five years old – cannot accommodate a new vision, perhaps we can expect some radical surprises in the 1999 Performance Index festival giving us a measure in a field especially marked out as open, flexible and ready to include risks.

Linda Cassens

NOTES

[1] I have borrowed some of these fabulous terms from Charles Bergengren's and Holly Morrison's 'Certain Uncertainty: The Cleveland Performance Art Festival', in *P-Form*, Number 43 (Spring/ Summer 1997), pp. 11–18.
[2] 1999 CH Performance Netzwerk: 28–29 February, *Die Schwarze Lade*, Boris Nieslony , Pfäffikon; 7 March, *Performance Conference*, Glarus; first two weeks of March, *Artist Laboratory* and 13–14 March, *Pow Wow*, Zurich; 26–28 March, *Performance Index Festival*, Basel.

INFORMATION

Performance Index
Haltingerstrasse 98
CH-4057 Basel
Switzerland
tel./fax 0041.61.692 .9451
email: pindex@thing.at
A preview of the archive on artists and events is available via:
http://www.thing.at/ performance-index

Performance Research: On Place

Notes on Contributors

THE EDITORS

Ric Allsopp is a joint editor of *Performance Research*. He is co-founder of Writing Research Associates, an international partnership organizing, promoting and publishing performance. He is currently a research fellow at Dartington College of Arts. He has been a research associate with the Centre for Performance Research since 1986, and has been associated with the School for New Dance Development, Amsterdam since 1990.

Richard Gough is general editor of *Performance Research*. He is senior research fellow in the Department of Theatre, Film and Television Studies at the University of Wales, Aberystwyth and Artistic Director of the Centre of Performance Research (CPR), the successor of Cardiff Laboratory Theatre, of which he was a founder member. He edited *The Secret Art of the Performer* (London: Routledge, 1990) and has curated and organized numerous conference and workshop events over the last twenty years as well as directing and lecturing internationally.

Claire MacDonald is a joint editor of *Performance Research*. She is a writer and critic and is currently completing a book on feminism and performance art for Routledge. She was head of Theatre at Dartington College of Arts 1987–9 and is now senior lecturer and research fellow in theatre at De Montfort University in Leicester, UK and a visiting professor in the Theater Arts Department, Mountholyoke College in Massachusetts. She was a founder member of Impact Theatre and Insomniac Theatre companies and has written performance texts and librettos for many productions, including, most recently, the script for the music theatre piece *Beulah Land* (London, ICA, 1994).

GUEST EDITORS – ON PLACE

Mark Minchinton has been a performer and performance maker for more than twenty years in many different contexts around Australia. He writes about performance practice and theory, and is a Senior Lecturer in Performance Studies at Victoria University, Melbourne. He lives in Footscray.

David Williams teaches in the Performance Studies program at the Victoria University, Melbourne. In Australia he has worked as director, performer and dramaturg, with Ex-Stasis Theatre, the Lightning Brothers, Chrissie Parrott Dance Co., Insomniac Theatre and Alison Halit. He has edited collections on the work of Peter Brook's CICT, and the Théâtre du Soleil (forthcoming from Routledge); he has also been a contributing editor to *Writings on Dance*.

THE CONTRIBUTORS

Linda Cassens is a performance artist and researcher based in Basle, Switzerland.

Aleks Danko is a visual artist who works in sculpture/installation and performance. Born in Adelaide, South Australia in 1950, he has exhibited widely in Australia and internationally. He currently lives and works in Daylesford, Victoria, Australia. *The Voice in the Garden Shed* is taken from *HIDING IN THE LIGHT: a light vision*, exhibited at Adelaide Installations – the 1994 Adelaide Biennial of Australian Art.

Rachel Fensham lectures in Drama and Theatre Studies at Monash University, Clayton. Her research interests are in feminist theory, dance, and contemporary performance. Her PhD was on 'gender and theatricality' in relation to the embodiment of the performing subject in circus and melodrama.

Mark Franko, dancer, choreographer, scholar, is Associate Professor in the Theatre Arts Department at the University of California, Santa Cruz. His books include *Dancing Modernism/Performing Politics and Dance as Text: Ideologies of the Baroque Body*. His article in this issue is part of a manuscript in progress: 'Dance and labor: performing work in the 1930s'.

Leslie Hill is a writer and performer whose work has been commissioned, performed and published in Europe and the USA, including work made for international performance seasons such as *Bad Girls* and *Jezebel*. She is currently a resident artist fellow in performance and multimedia at the Institute for Studies in the Arts, Phoenix, and senior lecturer in the Theatre Department at Arizona State University. She is co-artistic director of curious.com multimedia performance company.

Barry Laing is a performer, director and teacher who has worked in theatre and new performance contexts, including dance and visual arts. He has trained in Europe and Australia with Monika Pagneux, Philippe Gaulier, Theatre de Complicité, Anzu Furukawa and Pantheatre. He is the co-recipient of the 1997–8 Gloria Payten and Gloria Dawn Foundations Travelling Fellowship, which will be used to develop a new work in France in 1998. His most recent performance was *Rapture*, a solo work at La Mama Theatre, Melbourne.

Brigid McLeer is an artist and writer based in the UK. Her most recent installation was included in the group show 'Dark Field' (London) in June 1998. She is presently a lecturer in Performance Writing at Dartington College of Arts, UK. *Deixis ('absence of what qualifies the surface?')*, the pagework in this issue, draws on the idea of deixis (the phenomenon that elements in a language, e.g. spatial pronouns like 'here' and 'there', may have a reference which is dependent on the immediate context of their utterance) and the quote in the title is taken from Rachel Blau Du Plessis' poem 'Draft 21'.

Enrique Pardo, Peruvian-born theatre director, performer, writer and teacher, is director of Pantheatre (Paris) with Linda Wise, and of the Biennial 'Myth and Theatre' Festival. A member of the original Roy Hart Theatre group in the early 1970s, specializing in voice techniques, he founded Pantheatre in 1981. Pardo's most recent production, *Rosenhell und Bildersturm* (September 1997), a Bavarian macabre farce, is based on James Hillman's book *The Dream and the Underworld*.

Helen Paris is a founder member of the acclaimed Out and Out Theatre, Belfast, and currently working in residence at the Institute for Studies in the Arts, Phoenix, Arizona. Her most recent solo performance, *The Day Don Came with the Fish*, was commissioned by the London Filmmakers Coop and London Electronic Arts to open their new multimedia performance space, the Lux, in December 1997.

Karen Pearlman, a dancer/choreographer and a filmmaker/editor, is currently working on projects in narrative drama, documentary and video dance. She frequently writes about dance, her publications including various articles for *Real Time* and a book of essays, *New Life on the 2nd Floor* (Launceston: Tasdance, 1996). She is co-editor, with Richard James Allen, of *Performing the Unnameable: An Anthology of Australian Texts in Performance* (forthcoming from Currency Press and *Real Time*, 1998).

Mike Pearson is an Assistant Director of Brith Gof and Lecturer in Performance Studies at the University of Wales, Aberystwyth. He is currently co-writing a volume on points of contact between theatre and archaeology, and devising a series of performances with designer Mike Brooks on notions of place, memory, autobiography and personal narrative.

Zsuzsanna Soboslay is a freelance writer, director, lecturer, reviewer, performer and bodywork therapist who has worked along Australia's east coast and in Adelaide. In 1995, she received an Australia Council grant to study with butoh and shamanic teachers in Japan; in June 1997, at the invitation

of LIFT, she travelled to London as part of the writing team from *Real Time*. Her latest project is a dialogue with her daughter, due to be born in March 1998.

Peter Stafford worked as a professional musician in Sydney, before moving to Perth, where he now works as an artist/performer and lecturer/teacher. Recent work includes a number of Festival of Perth projects, as well as Fringe Festival exhibitions, installations and performances. More recently, he has been working on a series of street theatre events that address ecological issues. He is currently completing a doctorate in Fine Art and Performance at the University of Western Australia.

Nigel Stewart is Lecturer in Theatre Studies at Lancaster University, UK, where he specializes in dance and physical theatre. He has worked extensively as a director and choreographer, most notably with Theatre Nova, Triangle and Odin Teatret, and presently dances with the improvisation collective Grace & Danger. His researches into the body in performance are guided by an interest in the bearing between movement analysis and critical theory.

Nicholas Till is course leader of the MA Critical Studies in Visual Art and Theatre at Wimbledon School of Art, London. He practises as a theatre writer and director, and is author of *Mozart and the Enlightenment: Truth, Virtue and Beauty in Mozart's Operas* (London: Faber & Faber, 1992).

Clive van den Berg lives and works in Johannesburg. He lectures at the University of Witwatersrand in the Department of Fine Arts. He is interested in how and what we remember, the imaging of queer identity, and the role of public space in the formation of identity. His work is exhibited widely in South Africa and internationally.

Linda Marie Walker is an Adelaide-based writer, artist, curator and teacher. Her writing is widely published in art journals, as well as in literary journals and anthologies. Her first novella was published in 1989, and a second one will be available late in 1998. She is presently completing her PhD at the University of Western Sydney, Nepean.

Tracey Warr is a curator and critic who has worked with a range of international performance and installation artists over the last ten years. She is editor of *The Artist's Body 1945–95: A Source Book*, to be published in spring 1999 by Phaidon Press. She is currently a researcher at the Surrey Institute of Art and Design, and is completing a PhD on Earth Art.